CANCER DOCTOR

ALSO BY BARTH HOOGSTRATEN

Cancer Research: Impact of the Cooperative Groups

Breast Cancer (with R.W. McDivitt)

Lung Tumors (with B.J. Addis, H.H. Hansen, N. Martin, S.C. Spiro)

Breast Cancer (with I. Burn, H.J. Bloom)

Hematologic Malignancies

And the historical novel

Eyes of the Blind

CANCER DOCTOR

Barth Hoogstraten, MD

iUniverse, Inc.
New York Lincoln Shanghai

CANCER DOCTOR

iUniverse books may be ordered through booksellers or by contacting:

iUniverse
2021 Pine Lake Road, Suite 100
Lincoln, NE 68512
www.iuniverse.com
1-800-Authors (1-800-288-4677)

The names of the patients mentioned in this book were changed to protect their privacy. Any similarity to an actual name is unintentional and purely coincidental.

ISBN-13: 978-0-595-36010-9 (pbk)
ISBN-13: 978-0-595-67314-8 (cloth)
ISBN-13: 978-0-595-80461-0 (ebk)
ISBN-10: 0-595-36010-6 (pbk)
ISBN-10: 0-595-67314-7 (cloth)
ISBN-10: 0-595-80461-6 (ebk)

Printed in the United States of America

For Nienke;

our children: Frank, Evelien, Marion, and Nick;

my early colleagues, the true pioneers;

and our patients, the real heroes.

HOPE is the thing with feathers
That perches in the soul,
And sings the tune without the words,
And never stops at all,

And sweetest in the gale is heard;
And sore must be the storm
That could abash the little bird
That kept so many warm.

I've heard it in the chillest land,
And on the strangest seas;
Yet, never, in extremity,
It asked a crumb of me.

—Emily Dickinson (1830–1886)

Contents

FOREWORD

When at age ten, he was operated on for a large tumor on his ankle and a few days later the boy in the bed next to him died, Barth Hoogstraten knew that he would become a doctor. Eight years later, in 1942, he entered medical school in Nazi occupied Holland only to see his study interrupted when he was forced to go underground. In 1949, after lengthy military service in England and the Far East, he once again began medical school training. In 1956, he immigrated to the US and started an internship in a community hospital in Brooklyn not noted for its ties to academic medicine.

After two years, he moved to the Mount Sinai Hospital in New York City, a major academic health center, for training in hematology, a newer specialty with a flourishing science. This is where our paths intertwined. It was an era when the domination of cancer care by surgeons and radiation therapists began to be displaced by hematologists, who treated patients with leukemia and metastatic cancer with drugs, most of which had been developed and tested during WW II. The National Cancer Institute (NCI) created the Cancer Chemotherapy National Service Center that soon functioned as a pharmaceutical firm. It sought new agents (drugs) worldwide, tested these in its many laboratories and tried them out in the experimental animal and in man.

In 1956, the NCI developed the cooperative groups program that has contributed in a significant way to cancer treatment. It was as a leading member of these groups and as the chairman of the world-renowned Southwest Oncology Group that Hoogstraten made his major contributions to the science of cancer care. He chaired the subcommittee of the National Breast Cancer Task Force that developed the guidelines for the design of clinical trials and management of breast cancer. He served twelve years on the Current Treatment of Cancer committee of the International Union Against Cancer headquartered in Geneva.

As the title *Cancer Doctor* indicates, the major emphasis of this book is on cancer and on the pioneers with whom Barth was involved throughout his career. In his own inimitable way, he goes down the mainstream of his career and takes trips up side streams to delve into the details of his relationships with his fellow "cancer doctors." Very charmingly and often poignantly, he describes his role as a bedside physician in the care of individual patients and his interactions with them.

Hoogstraten's book brought back to me many memories of the time I sat on the sidelines watching the development of cancer chemotherapy.

Nathaniel I. Berlin, MD, PhD
Former Director, Division of Cancer Biology
and Diagnosis, the National Cancer Institute.

INTRODUCTION

Fifty years ago, in 1955, modern cancer chemotherapy was introduced by a handful of doctors who had only two not-so-good drugs with which to work. They had a seemingly never-ending enthusiasm, and the hope that they would one day successfully treat acute leukemia. I joined that small group two years later, and struggled through the many years of constant failures with them, the years when our patients—children and adults—suffered so much from this terrible disease and then died so bravely.

Who were those physicians who treated that seemingly hopeless disease? How could they face, day in and day out, the constant failures? Were they immune to the many deaths? Did their failures affect their family life? One of my medical colleagues once said, "You people must be a special breed to be able to stand losing all your patients. I certainly couldn't do it."

He hit the nail on the head. We were of a special breed, and initially, our ranks were thin. We were a rather disorderly bunch that tended to break the rules of clinical research, and create new ones. The constant failures made us insecure in many ways, and vulnerable to our own doubts. Not many hematology residents chose a career in cancer research after exposure to acute leukemia during their first year of training. In 1970, a former chairman of medicine at the University of Kansas said, "I never allowed cancer patients on my floors. These young doctors should not be exposed to something they can not treat anyway."

We were eternal optimists, and we never appeared depressed in front of a patient. Instead, we were uplifting, and full of empathy, warmth, and understanding. We gave until, at the end of the day, there was little left to give, until the barrel of giving was empty. Then, slowly, one child at a time, some patients began to respond, and a miracle happened: one child survived. We heard anecdotes of other children who lived five years and longer after they had learned of their diagnosis. Finally, we too were on our way toward success.

No longer is the outlook on leukemia, lymphoma, breast cancer, testicular cancer, and some other forms of cancer as hopeless as it once was. The treatment of cancer has come a long way since the middle of the twentieth century, but there is much still to be done. It will be many more years before people no longer fear learning that they have cancer, because they will have a chance. When present researchers have that feeling of hopelessness from time to time, let them remember the early pioneers who had nothing with which to work.

The inspiration for writing this book came from my colleagues, from the patients, and from my wife, Nienke, without whom I might not have made it. This book is unique because these individuals are included as equal partners in our battle. Cancer can bring out beauty, and a special understanding of life in all three, which is something I have tried to bring to the reader. It is my hope that they too will be richer, and remember what those few pioneers accomplished.

1

THE INSPIRATION

On May 13, 1924, I was born with a tumor on my right ankle. By the time I was six, that foot no longer fit into a shoe. Dad cut away the instep of a wooden shoe, and from then on, I wore *klompen,* as we say in Holland. The boys already called me all sorts of names for my red hair—even some grown men did that—now they added another one: "Clubfoot, clubfoot, the redhead has a clubfoot." I used to fight a lot. That tumor continued to grow, and finally my schoolteacher urged Mother to schedule a surgery to have it removed.

Nine days after the resulting operation, a nurse came with a tray full of bandages, and shiny steel instruments that looked like scissors, tweezers, and something that strongly resembled a very small, very sharp knife.

Dr. Huisman stopped by a few minutes later. "Well, young man, let's have a look." He began to remove the bandage, and I was scared. Bandages get stuck to a wound. It hurts when they come off, and I had a big bandage.

"You want to see your new ankle?"

It had not hurt at all. The big lump was gone, the six-inch incision looked ugly; there were many black sutures. Dr. Huisman removed some of them while I looked on. He only took the ones that moved a little when he tugged on them.

"The other ones aren't ripe yet," he joked.

Two days later, he was back, and removed another suture.

"Here, you try it," he said, but I hesitated.

"Go ahead; you can do it. I'll help you."

He showed me how to hold the tweezers with my left hand, and the scissors in my right hand. I grabbed the end of a suture just as I had seen him do, cut it on one side of the knot with the scissors, and pulled. It tickled a little when the suture slid out. That was on my tenth birthday and the day I knew I was going to become a surgeon. Several years later mother told me that Dr. Huisman had warned her that he could not remove the entire tumor without causing permanent damage to the ankle. He said that it could grow back, but it never did.

Something else left a permanent impression on me while I was in the hospital; I saw death for the first time. The boy in the bed next to me looked at me.

"Hi, I'm Karel," he said. "What's your name?"

"Barth."

He was older than I was, maybe two years older. He was pale and thin, and he lay very quietly. His pajamas were wrinkled, not like mine; I wore new pajamas.

"You need new pajamas when you go to the hospital," Mother had said. I never had such beautiful pajamas before. There was light blue with a red ribbon on the lapels.

"Are you sick?" Karel asked.

"No, I'll have an operation. Did you have an operation?"

Karel looked at me, fatigued. "No, I'm sick. There is something wrong with my blood. Are you scared, Barth?"

"Nah, they'll put me to sleep." I had no idea what surgery was.

Karel became very weak, and one day a priest did something with him that I didn't understand.

"What did the priest do with you?" I asked Karel.

"He gave me the Last Rites," he replied.

"What does that mean?"

"They think that I'm going to die."

I had to think about that for a moment.

"Are you scared, Karel?"

"No, I don't think so. I am going to heaven."

I still didn't understand, but I was afraid to ask more. Karel hardly said a word after that and the next day they put a screen around his bed. A nun sat with him all day, and at night, I could see her shadow through the screen. Two days later the screen was gone and his bed was empty. The nun's eyes were red when she made my bed. "Karel has gone to heaven," she said when I asked where he was. She blew her nose in a yellow handkerchief. Karel has stayed with me the rest of my life. I know now that he had acute leukemia.

Throughout high school I wore a green jacket that mother made from discarded velvet curtains at one of the estates where she worked as a seamstress. It had four pockets and a belt around the waist. The pants came from the Salvation Army. They were made of sturdy brown material, and there was a yellowish area just left of the fly. I hated those pants. In 1942, when I went to medical school, Mother emptied the jar she kept under her bed, and bought my first suit for eleven dollars and forty-four cents. Dad's friends and the rest of the family chipped in for a Leitz microscope in a light brown wooden carrying box.

Dad was a bricklayer and a plasterer. He and his brother were two of only five living master craftsmen in Holland. Few houses were built during the Depression and World War II, and because dad was his own boss, he wasn't eligible for unemployment benefits. He took odd jobs here and there, like building a fireplace or a garden wall. My older sister worked in a factory, and my younger brother was still in school.

Medical school did not last long that year. Every country the Nazis occupied had its traitors, and Holland was no exception. One of the most notorious traitors was retired General Hendrik A. Seyffardt. On February 4, 1943, he became the Deputy Commander of the Dutch Legion for the Eastern Front, and the next morning two members of the Dutch underground rang his doorbell.

"Are you General Seyffardt?" asked Jan Verleun, a twenty-three-year-old student.

"Yes I am. What do you want?"

Jan answered with two bullets into the traitor's abdomen.

The Nazis responded with raids on the universities and executed fifty prisoners, innocent people they held hostage for an undetermined length of time. They also forced all students to sign a loyalty oath in which they promised not to commit illegal acts against the occupying force, and to obey all laws and regulations put forward by the Germans. I refused to sign. Not long thereafter, they ordered me to report for deportation to Germany to work as a slave laborer. Mother cried, neighbors gave me fruit for the long train ride, and Dad shook my hand. "You know how to take care of yourself," he said. "You'll be back."

I walked in the direction of the railroad station, but halfway there I took a detour to 35 Rembrandt Avenue, the home of two middle-aged spinsters, Ann and Bets Frank. They were both blind from birth. Four times a week I drove Ann to the Institute for the Blind where she gave piano lessons. When the sisters heard that I had to go to Germany, they insisted that I go underground in their house instead. My parents did not know anything about this.

I could no longer use my identity card because the Germans had my name on their wanted list. Ann talked with the director of the institute, and that evening a mysterious man came to her house. He took my photograph and fingerprint and left without saying a word. A week later, a false identity card dropped in the mail slot of 35 Rembrandt Avenue. My new name was Ernst Eduard Stern, born on January 15, 1927, which made me three years younger. I chose the Jewish name in defiance of the Nazis. "An uncircumcised, red-headed Dutchman with a Jewish name—that'll confuse them," I told the sisters. G. van Veen signed the card, number A35/No. 626825. After the war, I learned that he may have been one of the most important resistance fighters in Holland. He was betrayed, and the SS executed him in the dunes of Holland. I still have the card.

The sisters taught me to act as a blind person. I walked through the house blindfolded, and learned to write Braille and read it with my fingers. We also sheltered a Jewish woman whose family had scattered for safety. I made a secret hiding place for her under the floor in case there was a raid on the house. We lived as a most unusual wartime family, but after a year, we too were betrayed. The Gestapo raided the house and caught the Jewish woman, who was hiding under her bed. They found some of my underwear, a pair of socks, and a letter from the director of the Institute for the Blind explaining that the carrier was blind.

"What about this?" the officer asked and he held up the letter.

When the sisters did not respond, the officer realized that they could not see the letter. "Why didn't he take this letter from the director of the Blind Institute with him?" he persisted.

"Oh that. That belongs to Ernst. He is a blind student who is living with us. Did he forget that again? He always forgets something." Ann said.

The officer may have had his doubts, but he was happy with his catch of the day. He threw the letter on the table and said, "You people are hiding a Jew."

"She is our maid," Bets protested. "We are not hiding her. How can we know that she is a Jew?"

"She just works here. We are blind, don't you see?" Ann added.

Even the German could appreciate that logic. A soldier came into the hallway with a large map of Europe on which I had kept the Russian front line up-to-date with pins. He handed it to the officer and the pins rattled on the floor.

"What are you doing with a map if you are blind?"

"That doesn't mean that we can't feel. We like to follow the progress of the victorious German army," Bets could not resist, but her sarcasm did not penetrate the thick German skulls. They left without arresting the sisters. The Jewish woman survived the concentration camp, and after the war she and her two children went to live in Israel; unfortunately, her husband died in Auschwitz.

Meanwhile, I had managed to escape and found my way to the railroad station. The sisters had a friend, Cor Zieren, who was an engineer in the coalmine Maurits in Geleen, a town in the south of Holland. I wanted to reach him. I approached a locomotive engineer who was wiping his hands with a piece of cloth. "Do you know my cousin Henk van der Velde?"

"I sure do. Hell of a water polo player." Henk was also a railroad engineer.

"I'm on the run. Can you help me?"

Dutch railroad workers were fiercely anti-German, and this man was no exception.

"Hop in." He closed the cabin door behind us. "Where do you want to go?"

"Geleen."

He scratched his head under his cap. "Geleen…that's a long way from here. What do you think, Gerrit?"

"I think we can manage that," said his partner.

After four transfers and four crews, I arrived in Geleen. The Germans needed all the help they could get to move the coal from nine hundred feet deep to the surface and Mr. Zieren had no trouble getting me a job. I even received an *Ausweis*, a German identity card that exempted the holder from working in Germany. I was now a fitter of diesel engines.

Liberation came on September 18, 1944, by a unit of the 78th Armored Field Artillery, 2nd Armored Division, VII Corps, First Army, by Corporal Andrew J. Tarnik from Canonsburg, Pennsylvania. He slept in my bed, signed the Ausweis, and wrote his address on the back. "Look me up when you come to America," he said. He married a Dutch girl. After the war, they went to live in Canonsburg, in the house he had left when he went to war. On Christmas, 2001, I cleaned out my desk and found the Ausweis with his address. I called him, and he still lived there.

"Is your name Andrew Tarnik?"

"Yes."

"And did you sign an important document in 1944?"

"What do you mean 'important document'? Who are you?"

"I am the owner of that document, and you slept in my bed after your outfit liberated Geleen."

"Wait a minute. Wait—let me think. Are you the fellow with the red hair?"

"Yes, I am, and I called to wish you a merry Christmas."

"Well now, this is a nice surprise."

From then on, we corresponded and reminisced on the phone. Andy, aged eighty-four years, died on Sunday, November 9, 2003.

Soon after liberation of the south of Holland, I volunteered for the army, went from Dunkirk to England in an LCT (Landing Craft Tank), and received an English officer's training. After the liberation of the rest of Holland on May 5, 1945, the army sent me to Indonesia for three years. Before we shipped out, I went to say good-bye to Nienke. In the winter of 1939–1940, as I put on my skates on the side of a canal, I saw her—a girl in a yellow sweater. A boy my age was helping her with her skates. I fell in love immediately. A year later, she walked into my high school class, and when the teacher began the roll call with Catharina Adama, she said, "Nienke…my name is Nienke." We prepared for the final exam together, and she had no inkling that I loved her. When she learned from mother that I was seriously wounded on July 8, 1947, she enclosed a photo with the letter. My hopes soared.

In May 1948, I was military commander in Eretan-Wetan on the North coast of Java, the place where the Japanese had landed. One day, while drinking a beer on my porch, I saw a native funeral procession walk by and that gave me an idea. I had the two volumes of Todt's *Atlas of Anatomy*, but had trouble visualizing where the muscles attached to the bones and how the arteries, veins, and nerves fit in. A skeleton would help. With two soldiers and a shovel, we went to the cemetery, selected an old grave, and dug up a skeleton. I washed the bones and put them out to bleach on low wall of the porch. Two days later three villagers approached the guard at the gate and asked permission to talk to the *toean besar,* or the Big Sir.

"Toean, the bones, my wife is worried." They kept a safe distance from the bones.

"Oh, you think that this is your wife's father?" I pointed to the skull.

"Can the toean please help us?"

I called for a shovel, and we walked to the cemetery. They went straight to the still fresh grave of her father. I handed the shovel to the husband, who gave it to the second man, who in turn pushed it into the hands of the youngest one, who could not refuse. He started digging. "Thonk" went the shovel on the coffin, and off ran the three men. The skeleton made the study of anatomy much easier, and five years later, I sold it to a young med student.

I returned to Holland in May 1949, and I started medical school all over again. Now—nearly fourteen years after first entering medical school in 1942—I had finally made it. I wanted to make a career in academic medicine and was on my way to America, where there were many more opportunities for me than in Holland. I had twenty-five dollars in my pocket.

2

THE SURPRISED IMMIGRANT

It was two o'clock in the morning, and most passengers in the big KLM constellation were sound asleep when the voice came over the intercom. "*Dames en Heren, dit is Uw kapitein.*" ("Ladies and gentlemen, this is your captain.") The man next to me looked up from his book and shook his wife. "*Marie, word wakker, er is iets aan de hand.*"("Marie, wake up. Something is going on.") The captain continued, speaking English.

"*Wat zei hij allemaal?*" Marie wanted to know, but before her husband could translate, the steward repeated the message in Dutch and in German. I looked outside. The small light at the wing tip seemed brighter than before, keeping an eye out, as it were. A blade of the outside propeller angled above the wing. The nearly full moon lit up a broad landscape of bulbous clouds below us. Anxious passengers talked, and stewardesses went about answering the many questions. My neighbor tried to reassure his nervous wife.

"*Je hoeft je echt geen zorg te make, Marie.*" ("You really do not have to worry, Marie.") He turned to me and said, "It's her first time in an airplane."

It did not take long for the captain to come back over the intercom. "Folks, this is your captain again. We are going back to Amsterdam."

"If we were already halfway, why the hell can't we go on to New York?" an irate American passenger behind us wanted to know, but no one paid him any attention.

"Ladies and gentlemen, arrangements have been made for passengers to inform their family and friends in New York City," the steward announced. "KLM has reserved rooms at the Amstel Hotel so that you can have a few hours of rest while we wait for another plane or a new engine. Also, upon arrival at Schiphol, all passengers will have free use of telephones to contact their families."

I hardly noticed the many announcements. It was December 31, 1955, and I was supposed to start a rotating internship at Beth-El Hospital in Brooklyn the next day. It would have to wait. I pushed the back of my seat down, stretched my legs, and relaxed all of my 152 pounds. My thoughts drifted to Nienke, to her last kiss when she saw me off from Schiphol. She had left our nine-month-old son Frank in the care of her mother in Hilversum. We knew that we would not see each other for at least a year. Leaving Holland had been her idea. Actually, she had made that a condition when I asked her to marry me. "We live only once, and I want to see more of the world," she had said.

Nienke had been born on Sumatra and lived in various parts of the Dutch East Indies until she was fourteen. Her father was born in a province of the Netherlands called Friesland and like most Friesians his last name ended with an 'a,' Adama. Friesians were proud people with a streak of stubbornness in them. The family made several long boat trips between Amsterdam and Batavia, renamed Djakarta after Indonesia gained independence, and Nienke could tell stories about Bombay, Port Said, and other exotic places. She lived in a land where she went barefoot most of the time and wore only shorts and loose, thin dresses. She ate rice with sambal and fruits with names I had never heard. She played with native children whose language she spoke fluently. She rode by car and on horseback to places where the native people rarely saw a light-skinned person. When she returned for good to Holland, her skin was a tropical brown, unlike the pale Dutch children who had never seen other parts of the world. She was as strange to them as they were to her.

In early 1948, soon after she completed her postgraduate education, she left for England, where she lived with David and Mary Wild. David was a chaplain at Eton College when World War II broke out and was attached as a chaplain to 4th Battalion Oxfordshire and Buckinghamshire Light Infantry. He volunteered to stay behind with the rear guard at Dunkirk and accompanied the British soldiers to prisons and work camps in Poland. The Allied and Axis powers routinely exchanged chaplains, but David stayed on with the prisoners. He was awarded the Military Cross for "devotion to duty" and Member of the Order of the British Empire for "devoted service in promoting the welfare and maintaining the morale of his fellow captives." He wrote a book, *Prisoner of Hope*, about his extraordinary experience.

David became a housemaster at Eton, and Mary had her hands full caring and feeding the young students. When she became pregnant, they sought help and found it in Nienke, who stayed with them throughout the pregnancy and the months thereafter. David arranged for her to spend some time on the Isle of Mull with the family of a retired navy captain. From there she went from one Scottish family to another, including a stay with Lady Hendry in Aboyne. She enjoyed the Highland Games in Ballater and Braemar, where the royal family roamed the grounds as well. When she came back to Holland, the country had become too small for her.

I returned from the Far East in 1949 and was immediately put in a military hospital, where she visited me. After my discharge from the army, I asked her to marry me and she agreed on that one condition—we had to move to another country. Leaving Holland was fine with me. I felt outside the norm in medical school. Most of my 1942 classmates had completed their education, including those who signed the infamous decree of loyalty to the German occupiers, and I was seven years older than most of the rest of the class. I had some catching up to do, and, when the opportunity came, we chose the United States as our new country. That opportunity came in 1954, when Professor Isidore Snapper gave a lecture at our medical school. He may have noticed a student with bright red hair in the audience. When the great professor left, that student stood at the door and said that he wanted to continue his study in America. "Write me when you have passed the doctoral examine and I'll see what I can do," he replied. He did; he wrote that a position for an internship had opened up in Beth-El Hospital.

The plane had started its descent over the North Sea. The main cabin had quieted down to a murmur of voices and stewardesses were busy collecting breakfast trays. That is when the second engine on the right wing decided that it had done enough work for the night and it too gave up the ghost, but not before emitting a stream of bluish flames. The woman closest to the ominous light screamed. The steward immediately came over the intercom. "It is just the after burn of the engine, ladies and gentlemen. Nothing to be alarmed about."

His soothing voice had the desired effect, but nobody needed to be told that the plane was now flying on only two engines—both of which were on the left wing—and that the captain had his hands full keeping the big plane reasonably level. An eerie silence fell over the cabin, interrupted only by instructions from the crew. I had a queasy feeling in my stomach; it was my first long flight too. We went straight in at the airport, and when those wheels touched the ground, and the plane slowed to a taxi, even the normally stoic Dutch applauded. The experience was enough for several vacationers; they went home, including Marie and her man. The rest of us went to the Amstel Hotel from which I called Nienke, who was still at home.

"You arrived," she said cheerfully.

"No, I didn't. I am back in Amsterdam."

"Barth! They didn't let you in?" She sounded alarmed.

My visa mentioned in small print that the United States Government at all times reserved the right to deny its holder entry into the country. That was her first thought, that I had been turned away, forgetting for a moment that it was impossible to fly back and forth within twelve hours.

"No dear, we had some engine problems and they decided to go back. Look, I am at the Amstel Hotel; why don't you come over for a few hours?"

I slept until Nienke knocked at the door. "KLM pays for it, so we might as well have lunch," I smiled.

Four hours later, she brought me to the airport for a second time. "This time I don't want to see you back," she said.

It was still dark when our plane landed at Idlewild airport. I couldn't sleep on the plane, and waited, bleary eyed, in the slow-moving line for passport control. The immigration officer, a black man with an enormous stomach, studied my passport, looked up, and smiled: "Welcome to the United States."

"Thank you."

Before looking for my luggage, I went to the men's room. Seeing a long row of urinals amazed me. Most restrooms in European airports have two urinals, but this one had fourteen. Then the man next to me put a hand on top of his urinal. There was a ring with a huge stone on a fat finger. I stole another glance just to make sure—yes, there was the ring, and the fingernails were polished. I washed my hands and looked around for a towel holder, but there was none. Instead, I saw a man push a knob on a box against the wall and turn his hands under a nozzle. Moreover, the man with the ring and the nail polish zipped his fly up when he was finished. I still had buttons. This was a new country alright.

3

BETH-EL: A CRUMMY HOSPITAL IN BROOKLYN

The taxi dropped me off at Beth-El Hospital at the corner of Linden Boulevard and Rockaway Parkway. The night manager looked up when I approached his desk.

"Can I help you?"

"Yes please. My name is Hoogstraten."

"Oh yes, doctor, we were expecting you yesterday. Did you have a nice trip? Let me see now, you start on GYN in half an hour. Why don't you have some breakfast in the cafeteria and I'll take care of your luggage. By the way, where is your luggage?" He took a breath.

"This is it." I pointed to my small suitcase.

"That's all you brought with you?"

He shook his head in disbelief and directed me to the cafeteria. On the way, I suddenly realized that he had addressed me as "doctor." I would still be "mister" in Holland. "Doctor," had a nice sound to it. The black woman at the cafeteria laughed when I asked for bacon and eggs.

"You won't find bacon in this place. No sir, no bacon, not in this place. No sir."

Okay, no bacon. I was too sleepy to argue with her.

Doctor Silver, the chief GYN resident, met me in the doctor's lounge in the operating suite. Army-green lockers lined the walls, the carpet was pockmarked from cigarette burns, and discarded scrub suits were scattered all over the place. Two couches that had long ago seen their best days flanked a table loaded with partially empty coffee mugs, several of which doubled as ashtrays. A man in a scrub suit slept in the only easy chair. Silver kicked his legs.

"Get your butt out of here."

The man peered at Dr. Silver, pulled himself up, and grunted, "One of these days they'll get chairs for the orderlies."

Silver looked at me. "You're a day late doctor. You are scrubbed at eight, but first I want you to do an LP on Mrs. Bornstein in 215."

I said something about plane trouble and asked, "What is an LP?"

Dr. Silver frowned. "A lumbar puncture. You know how to do one don't you?"

"Sure."

"Well, you'd better get dressed."

He sank into the just-abandoned chair and shut his eyes.

In medical school, I had seen one demonstration of a lumbar puncture. The neurology professor stood on the floor of the amphitheater; meanwhile I sat on a bench on the top row, thirty feet up, not exactly in an ideal spot to observe the details of the delicate procedure. Thus far, all my medical learning had been from lectures, demonstrations, and books. I had never even touched a patient in medical school. That only came after the doctoral exam. Dutch medical schools did not have internships. Instead, they had a two-year externship during which the young doctors lived outside the school. They came to the hospital early in the morning to receive practical education and left late in the afternoon. Since I had to do an internship in the States anyway, I decided not to waste those two years and left immediately after the doctoral. I anticipated that I would have some problems in an American hospital, but a lumbar puncture fresh off the plane? The thought of asking someone else to do the LP never crossed my mind, but at least I had enough sense to ask an anesthesiologist for advice.

"That's easy," he said. "You put your left index finger on the spinous process and slide the needle over your finger in the direction of the navel. When you feel a slight give, you're in."

"Thanks."

"Good luck!" He didn't stop me.

On my way to room 215, I had visions of a two hundred-plus pound Mrs. Bornstein, old and with a crooked spine. Instead, she turned out to be a cheerful middle-aged lady; she was barely one hundred pounds, and she had the straightest spine for which a doctor could wish.

"Good morning, Mrs. Bornstein. I am Dr. Hoogstraten, and I'm here to do your lumbar puncture."

"You're German," she said. "Such a nice accent."

"No, I am Dutch."

"From Holland. I like the Dutch," she smiled, but her eyes said that she was worried. "Have you done many of these?"

"Quite a few," I lied. What else was I to say, "No, this is my first one," and scare the wits out of her? I put a chair next to her bed and put a pillow on top of its back.

"There now, you sit on the side of the bed and put your feet on the chair. Put your arms on the pillow and rest your head on your arms. I'll be working from the other side of the bed and I'll tell you exactly what I'm doing."

As I worked, I explained every little step.

"This'll feel a little cold," I said before cleaning the skin with alcohol and iodine solutions. I put sterile towels around her buttocks.

"Now you'll feel a little stick for the anesthesia."

While the procaine did its work, I prepared the trocar, the manometer, and the test tubes, and asked her innocent questions about her family.

"Now you'll feel some pressure."

The spinal trocar is a hollow 1/8-inch-thick steel tube; a sharply pointed rod fits neatly in it. After going through the skin, I pushed the trocar in the direction of the navel, very delicately, and there it was, the slightest give. It meant that the rod had punctured the membrane of the spinal canal. I pulled the rod out, and clear fluid appeared. I was in.

"How are you doing?"

A little voice said, "Fine."

An LP is always a scary procedure for patients, in large part because they can't see what the doctor is doing. A nurse should really have assisted me, but when I asked for one at the desk, I was told that no one was available.

"Well now, you're all done."

"All done? You mean it is over? I don't believe it."

"You better believe it."

I helped her back in bed. "I want you to stay flat in bed for the rest of the morning; otherwise you may get a headache."

"Thank you doctor. I really dreaded this. You must have done a quite lot of them."

Outside the room, I almost jumped with joy. "Man, you did it!" I punched the air with my fist. That morning we scrubbed on three cases, and, back in the doctor's lounge, Silver asked the other intern to take the night duty. "Barth had a rough time with his plane and all, and he looks pretty pooped."

"No way, I was on call last night," answered an indignant intern, and so I was on duty that first night. At lunch, I asked for milk or cream with my coffee.

"No sir. No milk and no cream. Only black coffee." It was the same woman.

"I always have milk or cream with my coffee," I said.

She chuckled. "No sir, not for lunch, not in this place. You just wait right here." She yelled something over her shoulder and soon a little man with a funny, shiny black cap on the back of his head appeared from the kitchen.

"Can I help you?"

"Yes sir, I like to have some milk or cream with my coffee."

"Well doctor, this is a kosher hospital, and we do not serve dairy products and meat together." He peered over his half glasses.

"What do you mean, kosher?" I had never heard the word before.

Patiently he said, "Beth El. It means house of prayer. This is a Jewish hospital." He did not explain further, shook his head, mumbled something that sounded like "*Oy vay*" and disappeared into the kitchen.

I knew that Jews only ate the meat from ruminating animals, but why not with milk? It comes from the same animal. The episode reminded me how little I knew about Jews. Holland had a Jewish population of about 140,000 before the war, among them 34,000 German refugees who we welcomed with open arms. Throughout the centuries, the Dutch have accepted refugees without prejudice. The Jews from Spain during the sixteenth century, the Huguenots from France, the Pilgrims from England, and the Queen even gave Kaiser Wilhelm a place to live after World War I.

Our town, Hilversum, had about six hundred Jewish families. They lived amongst us without questions, without finger pointing. Jacob and Nathan Cohen were two of the best soccer players in town, and when Nathan once scored that winning goal during the second overtime period the whole town rejoiced. We were the champions. I remember the synagogue with the heavy double doors and the arched widows. When mother became deathly ill with a gastric hemorrhage, Dr. Sal Zwaap rushed over on his bicycle in the middle of the night and saved her life. David Lopes Diaz, whose family escaped from Spain in the 1580s, was elected town counselor for twenty-one years and council member for thirteen years. Why not? They were Dutch.

Dr. Zwaap was a pillar of strength for the Jewish community. Salomon Zwaap was born in Amsterdam on January 31, 1906, the son of Levie Zwaap and Roosje Goudsmit. He was a youngish looking man with fiery red hair, just like mine. He married a beautiful coloratura singer, Ester Philipse, and they had two children. The Zwaaps wore the yellow Star of David with great dignity. When the Jews were ordered to report for internment into a camp, Sal Zwaap came to say a last goodbye to mother.

"You know you don't have to go, don't you?" mother told him. "We and others will give you and your family a safe hiding place."

"Thank you Mrs. Hoogstraten, but I have to go," he replied quietly. "My people will need me," and he left.

Sal Zwaap made the greatest offer a doctor can make: his life. He went not only as a physician but also as a Jew, with pride in his people and a deep feeling of destiny. Judaism teaches that no man shall separate himself from his community, and Dr. Zwaap, a deeply religious man, wished to stay with his community of Jews to better overcome the evil of the Nazis. He became part of Jewish history.

The Dutch Civil Registry is unbelievably thorough, and so today we read under number 372 of the Registry in Hilversum the following entry: "Today, May 8, 1951, I report as official of the Civil Registry of Hilversum, that based on a report from the Ministry of Justice, on October 1, 1944, died in Auschwitz, Poland: Zwaap, Salomon, age 38, no occupation, born in Amsterdam, lived in Hilversum."

No occupation, it cries. Of our 600 Jewish families, only 40 returned at the end of the war.

After lunch, I crossed the road to one of two dilapidated houses for the interns and residents and inspected my room. Pieces of plaster hung from the ceiling, faded wallpaper torn in several places, cobwebs in the corners and a tear in the curtain. The mattress on a white, steel-framed bed sagged, and a naked light bulb hung from the middle of the ceiling. A straight chair, a small table, and a telephone completed the furniture. The woodwork had not seen a paintbrush in decades. The closet was barely large enough for my few clothes. There was a washbasin in a corner, but the hot water tap did not work. The toilet and shower were down the hall. The basement of the building next door served as the entertainment center for the house staff. It came complete with a table tennis set on wobbly legs, three bats with most of their surfaces long gone, a small black and white TV, an empty refrigerator, and cockroaches. A cleaning lady came by once a week to change the linen. This dreary place was to be home for the next year or so.

That evening I admitted eight new patients, took their histories, did complete physical examinations, and drew their blood. One patient, a thirty-four year old woman with the admission diagnosis of fibroids of the uterus, was scheduled for a hysterectomy the next morning. Her swollen breasts, dark nipples, and the bluish hue of the vulva were a dead giveaway that she was pregnant, so I called her doctor at home.

"Sir, I think that Mrs. Cohen may be pregnant."

There was an explosion on the other end of the line. "Who the hell do you think you are telling me what my patients have? What the fuck do you know about GYN?"

"Sir, I don't know when you last examined her, and I thought you might not know about a possible pregnancy."

"I know damn well that she isn't pregnant. From now on you stay away from my patients, you hear."

"Yes sir, loud and clear." I learned that expression in the army.

It was well past midnight when I hit the sack. Fortunately, I was only called out of bed twice. The next day, I assisted with the surgery of Mrs. Cohen, and she did have one small fibroid. The surgeon did not know whom I was and was even less interested in finding out. He did not open the uterus when he finished. While I cleaned up, he must have said something to Dr. Silver about last night's call.

"Let me give you a piece of advice, Barth," Silver said when I came into the lounge. "When you disagree with the admission diagnosis, tell me about it, and I will handle it. Never, ever, call the private physician at home if you want to stay out of trouble."

I checked in pathology that afternoon and there was a fetus. Two days later a pathologist wrote in his report, "The specimen is a uterus with multiple fibroids."

The second day I paid my respect to the grand old man himself, Professor Dr. Isidore Snapper. At age twenty-nine, this remarkable man became the youngest-ever professor of medicine in Holland. By that time, he had already written a scholarly essay on bone diseases. Throughout his distinguished career, he continued to study his favorite disease. The book *Multiple Myeloma* by Snapper, Turner, and Moscovitz became a classic. The authors described several previously unknown aspects of the disease.

When the Nazi Party won the 1933 election in Germany, Snapper saw the writing on the wall. He left Holland to become a professor of medicine in Shanghai. From there he moved to the University of Chicago, where, as chairman of the Department of Medicine, he formed a famous duo with another giant, Professor Hans Popper, the chairman of pathology. Thanks to Hitler, Professor Popper had left his beloved Vienna and became an expatriate, as well.

Many stories made the rounds about Snapper, but the best—and the one he liked most,—had nothing to do with medicine. In his youth, he was a star soccer player in Holland, and when his playing years were over, he became an international soccer referee. His soccer experience came in handy one day in Chicago when a small-time hood, who had said something like, "Your money or your life," accosted him. Before the youth could finish the sentence, though, Snapper kicked him so hard in his crotch that he ruptured the thug's urethra (the canal leading from the bladder). Snapper then took the poor fellow to the emergency room for treatment and pressed no charges.

I brought him a box of Dutch cigars, Schimmelpennincks.

"Thank you, but I don't smoke. Give them to someone else," he said with the no-nonsense directness for which he was well known—and feared—throughout his long career. He was an imposing figure, six feet tall, with the weight of a successful older man and a large head with a sunburned dome. Beth-El was a second rate, maybe even third-rate hospital, and Dr. Snapper, at seventy-plus years, was well past his heyday. From Chicago he and Hans Popper had moved to Mount Sinai Hospital in New York City, where they continued to star at the weekly CPCs, the Clinical Pathological Conferences. When Snapper reached the mandatory retirement age, he looked for another place where he could reign as king, and Beth-El welcomed the famous man with open arms.

"Work hard and you'll make it," he advised me. "This is a great country, with lots of opportunities, but if you want to make something of yourself, you have to work twice as hard as your American colleagues. Good luck." He returned to the book he was reading when I had come in. It had been a short interview indeed.

Gynecology, or GYN, was a surgical service, and I loved every day of it. I collected pieces of discarded sutures from the operating room floor and at night practiced making knots on the foot of my bed. By the end of the month, the white frame was black with sutures, and I could make knots with my eyes closed. One surgeon took the time to teach the interns. He let us feel the warm organs in the abdomen, the cyst, the tumor and the fibroids. Medicine had come alive. Dr. Silver showed me how to make a Hollywood stitch—put a continuous suture just under the surface of the skin, pull on both ends, and the edges of the wound come together so that you can hardly see the incision.

My next month of service was obstetrics, or OB, and I blew it a second time. In Beth-El, every woman had to have an epis, short for episiotomy, which is an incision through the muscle layer between the vagina and the anus. It is supposed to minimize the risk of a tear in the wall of the vagina during the delivery. This procedure was seldom performed in European hospitals at that time. On day one, I assisted the chief OB resident, and the baby's head came just when he started with the epis.

"Hold that head back," he ordered.

I put my hand on the head of the baby.

"Hold it!" he yelled. "Hold it! Goddamnit, now look at what you've done."

I hadn't done anything. Ever try to hold a baby back with one hand, while the mother pushes it out? That head was coming no matter what. The patient was a big woman, and with her powerful contractions that baby was going to be born right there and then, no matter what the resident said.

"Damn it, now what am I going to tell her doctor? He'll be madder than hell."

The resident was really pissed, but the woman had already given birth to eight other children, and her birth canal was so wide that this baby sailed through with the ease of a pleasure boat going through the Panama Canal.

"Come on, Joe. You know as well as I do that this woman didn't need that epis. What's all the fuss about?"

"I promised her doc an epis, that's why." Joe was still steaming.

Just then, late as usual, the family physician hurried into the delivery room while putting a scrub jacket over his shirt and tie. He hadn't bothered to cover the rest of his clothes, not even his shoes.

"What the hell is going on, Joe?"

"I'm sorry doctor, but there was no time to complete the epis. She came too fast," Joe took me off the hook.

"Oh shit, let me see." He ducked under the sheet where Joe and I had been working and looked at the wound.

"Wait a minute. You did make the incision." He sounded relieved.

"Only through the skin, not deep enough to call it an epis," Joe said.

Nevertheless, it was enough for the doctor. "You still have to put in a few sutures, don't you? And she'll feel them tomorrow, won't she?"

Joe shrugged his shoulders and put in three sutures while the doctor waited.

"Okay, Saul. Wake her up."

The anesthesiologist, who had remained oblivious to the affair, turned a few valves. The woman came slowly around as her doctor hovered over her, holding his scrub suit closed at his neck so she could not see his tie.

"Hi honey. You have a baby boy, and everything went fine."

The patient managed a faint smile, and the doctor, knowing that she had seen him, left the delivery room, calling over his shoulder, "Come on, Joe. He can clean up." "He" was I, whose presence he had not acknowledged until then. The doctor had already left when I entered the lounge. Joe was in a good mood as he made a note in a little black book. "He paid anyway, but remember one thing from now on. No matter how easy it is going to be, when they have a private doctor, the patient must have an epis."

"Why?"

"Easy. I knew that she didn't need one, you knew, and he knew. But with an epis, he can charge more because it is a surgical procedure, and when he charges more, I get paid more for doing his job."

That was my first lesson on OB in Beth-El. All you needed was a patient, a baby, a chief resident to perform the delivery, and a private physician in a hastily thrown-on scrub suit. The chief resident kept a record of how much each doctor paid, and when he completed his residency, he turned the little black book over to his successor. When a private doctor did not pay, he would regret it.

That happened two weeks later when a family physician delivered a full-term fetus that had died while still in the uterus. Without asking Joe for help, he tried to repair the episiotomy himself, but as happens quite often in the case of a dead baby, the bleeding wouldn't stop. Instead of taking his time to look where the blood was coming from, he kept putting in suture after suture. The assisting nurse had seen enough.

"That doctor needs help," she told Joe as she came into the doctor's lounge, but Joe didn't budge.

"Go have a look what's going on," he ordered me.

The epis was one big ugly black mass of sutures through which blood oozed. The doctor was sweating profusely, and his hands were shaking.

"Please ask Joe to help me," he begged.

I left to fetch Joe, who was waiting with a grin on his face. The doctor stepped aside almost deferentially when Joe took over.

"You made a goddamn mess of it, didn't you?" Joe removed the mass of sutures, tied the still leaking blood vessel, and neatly put the tissue back together. If anything, he knew his job. They left the room together, and, as usual, I cleaned up while Joe wrote another name in the black book. The doctor had learned his lesson; pay me and I'll help you when you are in trouble, or, do not pay and you are on your own from now on.

Soon thereafter, I made trouble again. It happened when I was on call one night. A good-looking woman with light-blond hair was anxious about the delivery of her first baby. Her name was Ingrid, and she was of Norwegian decent, which made her one of the few patients at Beth-El who was not Jewish, Black or Puerto Rican. It was a quiet night for a change. The only other patient was admitted for observation, and I sat with Ingrid explaining what she could expect. She had already insisted on general anesthesia.

"Do you have children?" she asked.

"Yes, we have a boy, Frank."

"Did your wife have general anesthesia."

"No, she had a natural childbirth with the help of a midwife."

Ingrid was amazed. "No doctor and no anesthesia?"

"No. Nothing. Very few women in Holland have any anesthesia at all."

"But what about the episiotomy? Don't tell me that she didn't have local anesthesia?"

"No episiotomy either. When Frank's head appeared the midwife carefully massaged the vulva over his head and out he came. I still remember Nienke's happy face when it was over. She wanted to experience all of it."

"Nienke, what a nice name."

She was quiet for a while, and I left the room to check on the other patient. When I came back, she said that she also wanted a natural delivery, without anesthesia.

"Well, you better first talk that over with your doctor."

Her obstetrician tried to talk her out of it, but she insisted. He and the anesthesiologist were furious and afterwards accused me of interfering with their business. They complained to Dr. Levine, the director of the OB-GYN service, who called me into his office.

"Look, I don't give a damn what they do in Holland. Here we do it our way, and you stay out of it, or I'll kick you off the service. Capeesh?"

I had no idea what that meant, but I got the message. A week later Ingrid sent me a package with a little jacket for Frank and a note: "Thank you. I wouldn't have missed it for anything."

One of our duties as interns was doing the circumcisions on newborn baby boys. It was a simple procedure, complicated only by the fact that there was not much to work with. It brought me in contact with rabbi Twersky, who personally performed all circumcisions for the members of his synagogue, and he did it the old-fashioned way, with a stone knife, often at the home of the proud parents. I had envisioned the rabbi to be a wise old man with a white beard, curls in front of his ears, a long black coat, and black hat. Instead, he turned out to be a much younger man, with a flowing red beard and red hair that even the big black hat could not completely hide.

David Twersky was born in 1922 in Kishinev, the capital of the Russian part of Moldavia. The city, which is only forty miles from the Rumanian border and straddles the Byk River, had a population of 130,000 of which forty percent were Jews. David came from a long line of leading rabbis in Kishinev. In 1922, his father, Yitzchok Twersky, moved to New York, where he established the first

Hassidic synagogue in Borough Park, Brooklyn. David was only nineteen when his father died, and he took over the leadership of the Skverer dynasty of Hasidic Judaism.

The good rabbi ruled his flock with an iron hand. However, he cared deeply for every member of his congregation. Women especially depended on him. It was said that a woman would not buy a new coat without consulting the rabbi first. When a member of his flock was a patient in the hospital, he always found time for a visit. Doctors went out of their way when they learned that their patient was one of his because Twersky could exert great influence over their practice. Twelve years later, I witnessed another example of his dedication. I was working in Mount Sinai Hospital and already an expert in the treatment of Hodgkin's disease when I received a call from a woman who identified herself as calling from Rabbi Twersky's office in Brooklyn.

"The rabbi would like you to see Mr. Schlumer in room 516 in consultation."

When I went to see the patient, John Boland, the chairman of radiotherapy, was already at the bedside. We looked at each other and laughed.

"Rabbi Twersky?" I asked.

"Rabbi Twersky," he said.

That is how the man worked; he selected the consultant, and he did not mind calling two or three at the same time, as long as his flock received the best of care. David Twersky died on February 2, 2001, in Mount Sinai Hospital. He was one of those rare individuals people talk about long after they are gone.

My next rotation was on the Orthopedic Service. Most patients with a fracture came to the emergency room, or ER, and, unless the patient had insurance, the Beth-El orthopedists did not come to the ER during weekends or at night. That was when the interns did all the work, because the resident-on call also let it be known that we were to wake him only when there was a complication. It was an exciting time for a young, aspiring physician. The winter of 1956 saw one of the heaviest snowfalls in the recorded history of New York City and that meant lots of fractures. The so-called Chinese fingers that we used to set broken forearms especially intrigued me. It consisted of four tapered, miniature fishnets made of thin steel wire with a rope at the end. The nets fitted over the fingers and, by pulling the rope through an overhead pulley, the nets automatically tightened over the fingers and pulled the arm up so that it hung down by its own weight. That was usually enough to bring the fractured ends of a forearm in line, and we were then ready to apply the cast.

Relieving the pain was particularly satisfying to patient and doctor alike. The pain receptors of bones are located in the periosteum, or periost, which is the strong fibrous membrane that covers the bone. When sharp bone ends tear a blood vessel, the blood begins to accumulate under the periost and forms a hematoma, which, because of the increasing pressure, pulls the periost even further from the bone, which in turn makes it more painful. The hematoma also pushes the ends of the broken bone further apart, making the pain even worse. When we stuck a needle in that hematoma and the blood came rushing into the syringe, the patient instantly felt less pain. After injecting some local anesthetic where the hematoma had been, we set the fracture and took another X-ray to check the alignment of the bone ends. We then applied the plaster and took a final X-ray to confirm the outcome of our work. It felt so good to see the reaction of both patient and family when the job was finished. Sure, I was tired, but this was what it was all about. It reminded me of my ankle and Dr. Huisman. Now it was my turn.

We did not touch the compound fractures, the ones with the ragged bone edges sticking through the skin. That was the job for the resident or, in severe cases, for the orthopedist on call. Every morning, except on weekends, the attending staff made the rounds, starting in the X-ray Department, to view the films of the patients who were admitted overnight. Pity the intern when the films showed a poor alignment. It meant that the cast had to come off, the bone reset, and a new cast applied. Of course, that would not have happened if the attending physician had come to the hospital in the first place, but that was not the policy for non-private patients. They could not pay.

Without friends, I became lonely and somewhat miserable. Working day and night kept me from thinking too much about Nienke and little Frank, and I set my mind on earning as much money as possible and saving every penny until I had enough to bring them over to the United States. My salary was $100 a month; I had a bed to sleep on and three meals, five days a week and on weekends when I was on call. Now and then, the other interns offered me fifty dollars to take their place, and I took it. On the weekends that I was not on call, I stuffed my pockets full with sandwiches while going through the Saturday morning breakfast line, enough for lunch and dinner that day. Sunday lunch and dinner consisted of packages of saltines that I bought at the corner drugstore and ate in front of the television set in the basement, alone.

The director of radiology, Dr. Zimmer, gave me another chance to make some extra money. This enormously fat man with advanced liver cirrhosis—the result of many years of heavy drinking—was a friend of sorts. He taught me how to read X-rays.

"Can you take the calls for radiology on the nights that you are not on call?" he asked me one day. "I'll pay you $37.50 a month." It was a pitiful sum, but I grabbed it and, during the next seven months, I took and read X-rays at night. I made an extra $ 262.50 during that time.

After orthopedics came two months on internal medicine, which meant not only hard work and long hours but also superb teaching by Professor Snapper. The chief resident, two assistant residents, and six interns met every morning at the office door of the great man and, at eight o'clock sharp, he appeared, flanked by his two carefully selected assistants. Like a general, he swept through the corridors on the way to the conference room. His troops followed close behind. On the third day, he did the unimaginable when he found the room already occupied by the OB-GYN staff. Snapper walked up to Dr. Levine and said just one word: "Out!" Whereupon Levine and his staff walked out without even the slightest protest.

"The bastard," mumbled Dr. Silver when he passed me on his way out.

"That's the old man for you," the resident next to me said from the corner of his mouth.

That particular morning began with the presentation of a woman with a low-grade fever and vague abdominal pain. We had all examined her and could not put our finger on anything. The X-rays were negative and the blood chemistries were normal. This was just the kind of patient with whom Snapper was at his best. Nobody could examine a patient as he did. He moved his big hands slowly over the abdomen, tapped gently, and looked up. "This patient has pus in her abdomen." Not just fluid—no, it was pus.

We all knew that there was no fluid in the free spaces of her abdomen. Free fluid flows to the lowest points, and when the patient lies flat on her back, the fluid causes the flanks to bulge out. We called this a frog belly, and our patient did not have one. We had also taken X-rays with the patient lying on her back, on her sides, and standing upright. Even a small amount of fluid would have shifted to the lowest point, but there was no fluid on any of the films, so we were confident that she had none.

"Tap her," Snapper ordered the chief resident. He did, twice—nothing.

Later that afternoon, when I went to check on the patient, I witnessed a remarkable spectacle. Assisted by several nurses, the patient lay face down between two beds; her hips and legs were on one bed, and her upper chest, shoulders, and head were on the other. Her naked abdomen was hanging down between the beds. Sitting on the floor underneath her was Snapper. He gently percussed the belly, stuck in a needle at the lowest point, and out came some blood-tinged, cloudy fluid. He got up from the floor with some difficulty and handed me the syringe. "Any fool can get it when there is a lot. This is the way we did it without those fancy X-rays. Remember that." He walked away, his back perhaps somewhat straighter than usual.

Snapper's reputation truly came to the fore during my second month on medicine, and this time I contributed in a minor way. Peter Mullhead was a thirty-eight year old little man with severe shortness of breath. His chest X-rays showed what looked like fluffy cotton balls throughout both lungs, as well as a marked enlargement of the lymph nodes. In addition, he had multiple kidney stones, and every day he painfully passed gravel in his urine. Snapper told him to collect his urine from the previous twenty-four hours in a large jar, and every morning Peter went to work. The head nurse had placed a small table at his bedside and, using an old-fashioned tea strainer, Peter drained his urine through filter paper. With a small letter scale, he meticulously weighed the gravel and entered the amount on a ledger. He then cleaned his tools and table and was ready for the next twenty-four hour shift. We did not think much of these rough estimates, but Peter did. The great doctor Snapper, the only doctor who was addressed as 'professor', the man he considered next to God, had impressed upon him the importance of his daily task, and he performed it diligently, inevitably with the tip of his tongue in a corner of his mouth. "This is my laboratory," he said proudly.

This was in a time when patients spent more days in the hospital, and when doctors could still learn a lot from patients. Mr. Mullhead's blood chemistries showed a very high level of calcium and a low phosphate level. We all agreed that he had sarcoidosis, a rare disease with a mortality rate between five and ten percent. It explained all his symptoms, as well as the cotton balls. However, in patients with sarcoidosis, the blood calcium is rarely so high that it causes kidney stones. Peter was started on intravenous steroids, and he soon began to improve. The cotton balls in his lungs became smaller, and the lymph nodes decreased in size. He breathed easier, and his blood calcium dropped to near normal levels. However, something still puzzled us; his serum phosphate level remained low, and that should not be the case in sarcoidosis.

Snapper had a long, private talk with the patient and learned something that all of us had overlooked. Peter had an identical twin and, two years earlier, that twin had undergone surgery on his neck in a hospital in South Carolina. Snapper jumped at it. He personally called the hospital and found out that the brother had an operation for hyperparathyroidism. Tucked behind the two lobes of the thyroid are four tiny glands, the parathyroids, which play an important role in regulating the metabolism of calcium.

"This man has an enlarged parathyroid gland," the old man announced during rounds the next morning. "We are going to operate."

He discussed the situation with the patient and explained that the only way for him to get well was to have the same type of surgery that his brother had. "Mr. Mullhead, your lungs were still bad, and this will be a dangerous operation. Think about it and let me know what you want to do." However, Peter had already made the decision. "Professor, you're the boss. If you think that I must have surgery, then let's do it."

Sure enough, during the exploration of the neck, the surgeon found one of the four parathyroid glands to be enlarged. He removed it, and we waited for the blood chemistries to become normal. They did not. Any normal doctor would now have rested his case, believing he or she had done all that was possible. However, that is not how true giants work.

"Are you sure that the other three glands are normal?" Snapper asked the surgeon.

"Yes, I am; they're all normal size."

Snapper secluded himself in his office for several hours, and, when he came out, he made a profound statement, "Mr. Mullhead has a fifth gland, and that one is enlarged."

"The surgeons only saw four," said one of his senior assistants.

"There has to be another one, and that one is hidden behind his sternum."

"You're crazy," the chief of surgery said when Snapper told him to operate again. "That's much too dangerous. The only way I can find a fifth gland is to split the sternum, and then he will not be able to breathe. It will kill him. I'm not going to do it."

The anesthesiologist agreed with the surgeon. He did not want to take the risk either. However, it took more than those two to deny the stubborn, strong-willed Dutchman. He was convinced that he was right, and he told Peter so. He could have saved his breath. "Dr. Snapper, I am in your hands."

"Mr. Mullhead, you can easily die on the table," warned Snapper.

The little man turned his head and lay quiet for a moment. The head turned back.

"That'll be better than a slow death. Please go ahead, Professor."

Snapper imported a chest surgeon and an anesthesiologist from Mount Sinai Hospital, and behind the sternum, they found a cherry-sized gland. Peter left the operating room barely alive, in severe pulmonary distress. Immediately after surgery, his blood calcium dropped to dangerously low levels. This was a time for nurses and doctors to excel. This nonpaying, uninsured patient had to make it. He became our obsession, and everybody put in untold hours to keep him alive. Two days after the surgery, I happened to read an article in the latest issue of the *Journal of the Mayo Clinic*. The authors described, for the first time, that the corticosteroids reduce the absorption of calcium from the intestines, which in turn lowers the blood calcium levels. Our patient was still on high doses of corticosteroids for the sarcoidosis. I immediately went to Snapper.

"Sir, corticosteroids decrease the absorption of calcium. I just read it in this journal."

Dr. Snapper looked at the article and smiled. "Looks like we better reduce his dose; don't you think?"

From that day on our patient slowly began to improve, and, after three and a half months in the hospital, Mr. Peter Mullhead walked out, surrounded by a happy and proud staff. We even took a group photo. And Dr. Snapper? In the quiet of his office, this once world-famous professor, the author of numerous articles and books, wrote an article about a single patient in a crummy hospital in Brooklyn.

The medical service taught me how to interview the patient, the fine nuances of a physical examination, and the relationship between the patient, the laboratory data, and the X-rays. It was only through carefully questioning the patient that the old man discovered that Mr. Mullhead had a twin brother, something all of us had missed. It was Snapper who found that little fluid in the abdomen because he took the time to look for it and used an unconventional method to tap it. Peter Mullhead taught us more about body chemistry than many other patients combined did. I learned to take the time with each patient. It gave me the feeling of being a detective searching for secrets and clues that could lead to a correct diagnosis in a puzzlingly ill patient. Professor Snapper not only had immense medical knowledge but he also showed us how his mind worked. Making the diagnosis where others had failed was all-important to him. The treatment he left to us. He opened a completely new world to me, and he was in large part responsible for me becoming a clinical investigator.

I still wanted to become a surgeon and looked forward to the next four months, all of which would be in the Surgery Department. That is where the real excitement is. An open abdomen with the colorful organs and glistening intestines, the lungs sliding under an exposed rib cage with each breath, the hands of the surgeons working deftly together, and the moments when one could cut the tension. The instant success followed by the reward of discharging a happy patient in a few days or weeks. It was a macho world peopled predominately with men of decision, of action—the cutting and putting things together again. In July, two women joined the service as assistant residents, and they too became macho. On surgery, the doctors were sure of themselves, and they walked like it. On internal medicine, they were unsure and asked questions. They walked slowly while talking, debating. It was a science.

Dr. Zucker was by far the best surgeon. He was heavyset, five feet seven, and he had a terrible temper. He worked with two full-time assistants, both already qualified surgeons, and he always occupied two operating rooms at the same time. One assistant prepared the patient short of the actual incision and then waited for his boss to finish the other case and take a bathroom break. The second assistant stayed behind to close the wound, write the post-op orders, and dictate the operating note, a synopsis of the procedure.

Dr. Zucker taught as he went along, worked at a fast pace, and berated his assistants.

"Why do you tolerate him?" I asked one of them while we waited.

"Because he is the best teacher around. I call this my year of self-imposed apprenticeship. A good recommendation from him will open doors for me later."

One morning I was holding the retractors at my customary place to the left of Dr. Zucker, and the assistant was on the other side of the table. The patient was an obese woman whose gallbladder, filled with stones, was tucked under the liver at an awkward angle, deep down in her huge abdomen. I stretched my neck and tried to have a peek over Zucker's shoulder. He turned to me and stepped aside.

"Here—look. This is the common bile duct, here is the cystic duct; this big vessel is the hepatic artery, and there is the cystic artery. I'm going to cut that artery and the cystic duct and then dissect the bladder from its bed."

The word cystic comes from the Greek word *kystis*, for bladder, and is only used for the gallbladder and the urinary bladder. Now that I had seen the operative field, he continued with the surgery. He put two clamps on the cystic duct and was ready to attack the cystic artery.

"Suture."

The scrub nurse handed him a long, straight clamp with a curved needle and suture at the end. Deep down in the belly he had trouble feeding the needle under the artery because the angle was such that he could not see the point of the needle.

"Pull harder," he ordered, but I was already pulling on the retractors as hard as I could.

"Can you see it?" he asked his assistant.

"Not yet."

Zucker tried again. "Now?"

"No."

"Shit." The scrub nurse wiped the sweat from his brow.

"There—I see it."

"Grab it," but when the assistant tried to put a clamp on the small point it got away.

"Goddamnit, why the hell did you let it go? How do you expect me to work with jackasses like you? You're wasting my goddamn time."

He stopped working while he was yelling, and my arm muscles began to twitch.

"Sir, you're wasting my strength," I interrupted.

The red-faced surgeon turned to me, thunderstruck. Burning eyes over the mask slowly softened, and he went back to work as if nothing had happened. He finished and left, but not before giving a last swipe at his assistant. "Why the hell don't you guys ever say something like that?"

They would not dare.

Cardiac surgery just emerged from the experimental stage in 1956 and Beth-El was hardly the place for it. Nevertheless, the hospital allowed it because it brought prestige and income. Dr. Simone, a cardiac surgeon at Mount Sinai Hospital, came over to perform the delicate procedure and I twice scrubbed on patients with stenosis of the mitral valve.

The left side of the heart consists of two parts; the atrium on top receives the oxygen-rich blood from the lungs and pumps it through the mitral valve into the ventricle below. The mitral valve is also called the bicuspid valve because it consists of two leaves. This valve is constructed in such a way that it lets the blood flow from the atrium into the ventricle, and when the ventricle contracts, the valve shuts and prevents the blood from going back into the atrium. Instead, it all goes into the aorta and to the rest of the body. A healthy mitral valve opens to about four to six square centimeters, but in patients who had rheumatic fever as a youngster, the valve gradually becomes thicker with fibrous tissue and calcium deposits. As a result, the leaflets of the valve become rigid, stenosed, and the valve can no longer open or shut completely. When the ventricle relaxes to let the blood in, some blood will stay behind in the atrium, and when the ventricle contracts some blood goes back into the atrium. As the condition progresses, the patient ultimately goes into heart failure. Only an operation can correct the condition, and in 1956, this was a so-called closed procedure because the surgeon does not open the heart itself.

Luckily, God has provided the atrium with an auricle, which sits on top of the atrium. It is called the auricle because it looks like an ear, and the Latin word for ear is *auris*. Nobody knows why we even have an auricle, but it is there, and it communicates with the atrium. The surgeon can use that auricle to reach inside the heart with his finger and feel the diseased valve. When I assisted at this operation for the first time Doctor Simone explained everything as he went along. Also scrubbed was the chief surgical resident, Dr. Mark Miller. Fortunately, I didn't have to hold retractors for this operation, because, Simone used a device that spread the ribs apart so he could see part of the heart. Unlike other organs that perform complicated jobs, such as digest food, produce bile, or, oxygenate blood, the heart is only a mechanical device. It is a pump. I was excited, but when I saw the heart through the opening between the ribs, I was not overly impressed.

"I first make a purse string suture around the base of the auricle," Doctor Simone began. The needle went in and out at the base of the auricle and dragged the suture behind it.

"I now hold my index finger close by, and Mark will use the scissors to cut the auricle off just above the suture line."

He nodded that he was ready, and the resident cut off the part of the auricle above the suture. Doctor Simone immediately pushed his finger into the opening, whereupon Mark pulled the suture tight around the finger so that no blood could escape. It was just like an old-fashioned moneybag with a string.

"I'll now try to break up the stenosis with my finger." Evidently, that wasn't easy.

"It's as hard as a rock." He wiggled his finger for another five minutes and stopped. "That'll have to do. Ready Mark?"

He pulled his finger out as Mark pulled the purse string tight behind it. The most delicate part of the operation was over, and the resident was allowed to complete the surgery. Unfortunately, the patient improved only slightly.

For the second operation, the team consisted again of Simone and Mark, while I stood as usual to the left of the surgeon. We assisted while Mark did the preliminary surgery until the heart was exposed.

"I'll take over," Simone said at that point.

Mark, who was in his last year of residency, angrily looked up at Simone.

"You said that I could do it."

"No I did not. You're not ready."

"You promised," his voice rose.

"Well, you won't."

"Then you can damn well do it alone."

Mark tore off his gloves and stormed out of the room. For a moment, Simone looked perplexed, and then he turned to me. "It looks like we'll have to finish it together," he said, very calmly. "Please go to the other side of the table."

"Me?"

"Yes, you can do it. You've seen us do it"

I shuffled to the other side of the table. We finished the operation together. With extreme patience—and as nice as he could possibly be under the circumstances—the surgeon took me through the operation step by step. It wasn't scary; it was something that had to be done. When it was time to cut the auricle, I could feel the living tissue give way to the scissors. That night the patient died because the valve couldn't close tight enough. Mark Miller wasn't even reprimanded.

A week later, there was another tragedy. Mancho Khilnany, a fellow intern from India, was scrubbed, and when he walked into the lounge there was blood spattered all over him, and his brown face was pale.

"What happened to you?" I asked.

Mancho fell into a chair, his chin on his chest. After a while he murmured, "You won't believe it. It was terrible." He was shaking.

"Well, take it easy. Here, have some coffee."

He slowly sipped the coffee and looked up. "The chest was open and I could see the heart pumping. Dr. Simone asked for a scalpel and, when the nurse slapped the knife in his hand, it slipped. The point fell right into the aorta where it takes off at the ventricle. Barth, blood spouted all the way to the ceiling."

"What did Simone do?"

"Nothing. He couldn't do anything. He just stood there and said, 'damn, damn' over and over again. It was awful."

The patient died on the table, and it was the last cardiac surgery performed in Beth-El for quite a while. That operation required a team of expert surgeons and nurses in a room fully equipped for emergency bypass circulation in case something went wrong, and Beth-El had neither.

The interns on the surgical service covered the emergency room on nights and weekends. Beth-El wasn't exactly in a well-to-do, quiet part of Brooklyn, and the police had their hands full, especially on weekends. One Saturday night I was called to see a twenty-six year old woman with a stab wound on top of her left shoulder, between her collarbone and the shoulder blade. The knife had just missed the major arteries and nerves, but had punctured her lung, which had partially collapsed.

"Tell me exactly what happened," I told her.

"An ice pick fell from the ceiling in my kitchen. The string must have broke."

"Ma'am, this wound was not made by an ice pick."

The police officer standing nearby interrupted, "Doc, she is lying."

"It was an ice pick. Honest."

"No it wasn't. An ice pick makes a round hole, and this one is not round."

"It was a pick." The woman clamped shut.

"Doc, forget it. She'll never change that story."

The officer shrugged his shoulders, wrote in his report "One ice pick fell from the ceiling" and left.

Another evening I saw a fifteen-year-old boy with at least twenty holes in his back. He was markedly short of breath, but as cool as a cucumber.

"What on earth happened to you?" I asked.

"Nothing."

"Look, if you want me to help you, you must tell me how you got these wounds."

"Some guys worked me over with a two-by-four full of nails. And that's all I'm telling you."

The chest X-ray showed a partially collapsed right lung and a left lung completely down. I used a system called underwater bottle drainage to expand the left lung. It consists of a pump and two large bottles partially filled with water. A rubber tube connects the pump to the first bottle, and another tube interconnects the two bottles. The second bottle also has a second long tube, which I stuck through a hole in the chest wall that I had just made. The pump started, air was sucked from the chest cavity and bubbled through the water, through the pump, and out in the room. The lung began to expand.

The boy was lying face down; he was severely short of breath and in pain. Two police officers and a detective questioned him. His parents implored him to answer the questions, but the boy remained mum. There was quite a crowd around that stretcher.

"Can this please wait until I'm finished?" I asked the detective.

"Doc, you don't know these characters. Believe me, this is the only time he may say something."

The officers continued to pester the boy while I worked. However, they were right, the boy didn't say a word other than, "Fuck off." He was as hard as the nails that had put the holes in him. After the exasperated police left, the boy turned to me and said, "Thanks doc. I'll take care of them myself." That was Brooklyn then. I dressed his many wounds, wrote a note in his chart, and told the nurse that I would be back in an hour.

Halfway down the corridor I heard the scream of a child, and I knew it—there was a cockroach in an ear. Cockroaches not infrequently find a way into the ear of a sleeping child or sometimes of an adult. The body of a cockroach slants forward, and, once it is in the ear canal, it cannot turn around. It tries to go deeper but is blocked by the eardrum, and when it hits that drum it causes excruciating pain. An inexperienced intern will try to grab the cockroach with forceps, but that only makes matters worse, because then the animal struggles even harder and the child screams louder. There was a very easy way to get rid of the cockroach.

"Are you the mama?" I asked the woman holding the child.

"Si."

"Manuella!" I called out.

Our Puerto Rican nurse was already on the way. "Si doctor?" she teased.

"Do your duty, you lovely lady of mercy."

She let go of a torrent of Spanish words and the mother smiled at me. Manuella held the child's head firmly while I put two drops of ether in the ear. Seconds later, the cockroach was sound asleep and I pulled it out with forceps. You only had to know how.

I never completed the four months on surgery, and I didn't really mind. Standing through those long hours at the operating table, especially during neurosurgery, I developed pain in my right ankle, the same one that had been operated on for a tumor when I was ten years old. However, that was not the only reason why I didn't complete the surgery rotation. The Korean War forced thousands of young physicians into military service, and suddenly Dr. Snapper found himself without medical residents. He acted immediately by pulling Mancho away from the X-ray Department, and he called me in for a little chat.

"Is there any chance that they also call you?" he asked.

"No sir, I already served during the war."

"Good. How do you like surgery?"

"Surgery is fine, sir, but I have trouble standing for long periods."

"How come?"

"I had a tumor removed from my right ankle when I was young, and now the same ankle hurts when I stand too long in one spot."

"Well, I can't say I'm sorry to hear that, because I need you in medicine."

"But what about surgery? I can't just walk out."

"Leave that to me, and, by the way, you and Khilnany will be assistant residents."

"Does that mean we'll also be paid the extra twenty-five dollars a month?" I asked.

"No, it doesn't. Giving a salary to the house staff is a lot of nonsense. You should pay for the teaching you receive as we did in my time. You start tomorrow."

End of conversation—it made no difference that the surgical department was now shorthanded or that its chairman vehemently protested. It was a done deal and Snapper had shown once again that he was the boss.

One of our more challenging tasks as assistant residents was to find an interesting patient for presentation at the weekly Wednesday Grand Rounds, which every private family physician and specialist in internal medicine was required to attend. The residents prepared a summary of the case from which Snapper presented the details without mentioning the diagnosis. The radiologist discussed the X-rays and then each doctor had to write a diagnosis on a piece of paper. We collected the papers, and, after the conference, Snapper gave each doctor a rating. Grand Rounds were always showcases of the highest quality and superb teaching. Snapper, the ultimate showman, was never reluctant to bend the truth if that increased the educational value of the presentation. One week I selected a fourteen-year-old girl with hereditary spherocytosis, a rare form of anemia. The red cells in that disease resemble small round balls, and under the microscope they look deep red. Normal red cells are flatter and thinner in the center than on the sides. This shape makes the cells pliable and enables them to sneak easily through even the tiniest blood vessels, especially those of the spleen.

Red blood cells normally survive about 120 days, when, just like an old person, they can no longer bend so easily, and they get stuck in the fine network of capillaries in the spleen and die. Hematologists refer to the spleen as the graveyard for red cells. The rigid, round blood cells in hereditary spherocytosis are not pliable and many fail to pass through the spleen and die prematurely. Because of the extra work, the spleen grows larger, and the patients become even more anemic. Their bodies try to keep up with the increased demand by producing more cells in the bone marrow, but even that will not be enough. In desperation, the body then tries to form extra bone marrow in places where one normally does not find it. That extra bone marrow can sometimes be seen on X-rays. I searched the literature and read somewhere that in a few patients the extra marrow appears around the teeth in the lower jaw, the mandible.

"Take an X-ray of the face," Snapper ordered when I told him about it.

"I already did, and it doesn't show," I replied.

"Find me the X-rays of a patient who has it," he ordered again.

Dr. Zimmer and I delved into the archives of the Radiology Department and, after several days, came up with a patient with sickle cell anemia who had been in a car accident. An X-ray of his skull and face showed the abnormal marrow expansion in the jaw. Never mind that it was a different diagnosis and that the patient was a man.

"Show them," said Snapper and the next day Dr. Zimmer put up the X-rays. "Here we see the X-rays of the face of this girl," Snapper said with great aplomb. "Notice the typical bone marrow expansion around the teeth of the lower jaw."

Only three of us knew better and the show went on.

Snapper was so powerful and such an autocrat that he did not even hesitate to order private physicians to obtain a consultation when he thought it necessary, especially those physicians who did poorly during Grand Rounds. I once admitted a fifty-two year old woman with the diagnosis of atrial fibrillation, a much too rapid and irregular heartbeat. The patient had noticed her irregular pulse and had called a cardiologist she had never seen before. Without examining her in his office, he told her to go to the hospital, and he called in the typical orders for atrial fibrillation.

When I examined her, she had all the signs and symptoms of an overactive thyroid. She was anxious, nervous, agitated and weak. Her thyroid was enlarged, she looked at me with a stare, and her eyes were bulging. I called the doctor at his home.

"Sorry to disturb you doctor, but I think that Mrs. Bergman is a hyperthyroid."

"No, she has atrial fib."

"Yes, but I think that is caused by her thyroid condition."

"Just start my orders and I'll take care of it."

"Sir, I think we should ask for a consultation."

"What do you mean a consultation? She has atrial fib. I have my boards in internal medicine and cardiology and I can take care of it." He was clearly annoyed.

I let it go at that. We knew the physician for his frequent wrong answers at Grand Rounds and it made no sense arguing with him. The next morning I presented the patient during rounds, and Snapper immediately told the physician to obtain a consultation. He refused, and the old professor simply took the patient away from him.

It was strange that this seemingly all-knowing man had so little interest in the diseases of the heart. We were never permitted to present a patient with an interesting heart disease at Grand Rounds. One morning I examined a patient in a six-bed open ward when a new patient suddenly made a funny noise and grabbed his throat. I dropped what I was doing and listened to his heart, but what I heard made no sense to me. A quick lead with the EKG machine revealed only steep up and down waves, something I had never seen before. Was it ventricular fibrillation? If so, the patient could be dead in a few minutes.

"Get me pronestyl," I called out to an overweight nurse who happened to pass by in the corridor. She turned around and slowly waddled to the nursing station.

"Run!" I yelled, and she ran.

While I continued taking the EKG, the patient desperately pointed to the drawer of his nightstand. It contained an old spectacle case, and I thought that he wanted his glasses, but he pushed the case in my hand. There was no time to argue so I put it in my pocket. By the time the nurse came running with the pronestyl, the patient was no longer responding. I gave him a large starting dose and worked on him the rest of the morning. When I met Snapper in the corridor later that day, I showed him the EKG.

"Make sure you get the autopsy," he said and walked on.

The patient survived. Four days later, I overheard him talking to his neighbor. "I gave that doctor some money. You know, you got to do that if you want them to work on you."

I managed to keep my composure. "Oh—Mr. Levi, I put your spectacle case back in your drawer," and left. The case contained no glasses, only a small sum of paper money. When I asked Snapper whether we should present the patient at Grand Rounds, he declined.

Once a week the house staff also had an hour-long teaching session with the old man. The interns selected the patient and the assistant resident advised them how to present the case and what to look up in the literature to back up their diagnosis. This time the patient had a rare and complicated disease, named after a Swiss pediatrician, Guido Fanconi, who had described the disease in the late nineteenth century. A second physician, Dr. De Toni, had contributed much to better understanding of the syndrome, and I told the intern not to forget to mention his name during the presentation because Snapper could be very touchy if you forgot to give full credit. So the intern began his presentation as follows, "I'll present a patient with De Toni-Fanconi syndrome."

When he finished his presentation, Dr. Snapper gave a brilliant discussion of this very difficult subject. It was customary after these sessions for all of us to escort the professor back to his office. That morning, at the door, he thanked the intern and then turned to me.

"Where did you study medicine?" As if he didn't know.

"In Amsterdam, sir."

"Why don't you ask for your money back?" and he disappeared into his office.

I was dumbfounded and deeply hurt, in part because he said it in front of everybody. Later one of his assistants consoled me. "Don't let it disturb you. He really likes you."

"He has a funny way of showing it." I was still hurt. "What was that all about?"

"The intern forgot to add the name Lignac. It is Lignac-De Toni-Fanconi."

I looked Lignac up in the library and, sure enough, some people added his name to the syndrome. Lignac turned out to be a Dutch physician. No wonder Snapper had been annoyed. However, so was I, and I spent that weekend in the library of the Academy of Medicine in Manhattan where I found that a Swiss physiologist by the name of Emil Abderhalden and a doctor Debre had also contributed to the better understanding of the syndrome and that their names were sometimes added.

At the next session, I introduced the new topic as follows: "After last week's discussion about the Abderhalden-Lignac-deToni-Debre-Fanconi syndrome, we now present..." It really could have made the old man angry, but—if anything—he was a good sport, and he smiled. This time, after the session, he invited me into his office for a cup of coffee.

4

DR. LOUIS R. WASSERMAN

It did not take me long to fall in love with hematology, the study of blood. Looking into the microscope at the sheer beauty of the cells and their wide variety of colors and shapes fascinated me. Most interesting were the white blood cells, because they come in such a wide variety. Each cell consists of a nucleus surrounded by a substance called cytoplasm, and these structures are contained in a cell membrane. In their earliest form of life, the cells are called blasts, which is derived from the Greek word for bud or sprout, *blastos*. After going through several stages of maturation in the bone marrow, the cells reach a mature phase and are released into the bloodstream. Patients with acute leukemia have blast cells that, internally, are slightly different from normal blast cells, enough so that it prevents them from maturing into normal cells. They are then called leukemic cells, and they eventually crowd out the normal cells in the bone marrow and find their way into the bloodstream.

I was particularly enamored of the plasma cell, with its beautiful azure blue cytoplasm. The nucleus, instead of being in the center of the cell, is usually off to the side, and the adjacent cytoplasm is of a lighter blue mixed with light brown. Plasma cells normally do not enter the bloodstream. They stay in the bone marrow, and, when they become malignant, they too can rapidly take over much of the marrow space just as the leukemic cells do. The patient then has multiple myeloma, the disease with which Snapper had made his reputation.

On January 1, 1957, Snapper sent me to Mount Sinai Hospital in Manhattan for three months, where Dr. Louis R. Wasserman was chairman of the Department of Hematology. It was the only hematology department in the country; all others were divisions within departments of medicine. Mount Sinai was one of the most sought-after teaching hospitals in the country and routinely ranked with Duke, Stanford, and Massachusetts General in the top four. Sinai, or as we sometimes referred to it, "The Mount Sinai Hospital at the Park" to distinguish it from what we considered to be the less-important Sinais in the country, is located between 99th and 102nd streets between Park and Madison avenues. The complex consists of multiple buildings, interconnected by a network of subterranean corridors that form convenient meeting places for physicians, house staff, administrators, students, and visitors. The support staff pushed numerous carts and stretchers through this maze, and at any given hour the traffic resembled that of Times Square on a busy day. The Hematology Department was located on the third floor of the Berg laboratory building, one of the lesser structures.

Dr. Louis R. Wasserman, or LRW as he was sometimes known, was a short man, built like a solid tree trunk. He appeared to have been born with a perpetual scowl and an almost threatening look. Many people were frightened of him because, when provoked, he could explode into a ferocious tirade that tolerated no interruptions and could last as long as fifteen or twenty minutes. However, he could also be very pleasant, and he was known as a generous and charming host. The man seldom really laughed; he grinned.

Before burying himself in research, Wasserman made a leisurely trip around the world, and he became especially fond of Indonesia and Indochina. After he was inducted into the army medical corps during World War II, the placement officer read his resume. "I see that you were in the Far East," he said. "Then you must be familiar with tropical diseases." He assigned LRW as an infectious disease 'expert' to the North African theatre. "I knew nothing about infectious diseases, but they had to put me somewhere," Dr. Wasserman used to say.

Soon after the war, he took a position with 1939 Nobel laureate Ernest O. Lawrence, director of the famous Donner Radiation Laboratory at the University of California, Berkeley. Lawrence played a prominent role in the Manhattan Project, the making of the atomic bomb. On Wednesday, April 25, 1945, his twelfth day in office as President, Harry Truman met with his Secretary of War, Henry L. Stinson, and learned for the first time about the Manhattan Project, or S1, as Stimson preferred to call it. Not only was the freshman president told about the bomb's capacity to end the war but Stimson also advised him that it was time to consider the future role of atomic energy. On his recommendation, Truman authorized Stimson to form a select committee to study that role, and, on Wednesday, May 9, 1945, the Interim Committee met for the first time in Stimson's office at the Pentagon. One of its eight members was Ernest O. Lawrence.

Wasserman became interested in the application of nuclear physics in medicine. He concentrated mainly on iron metabolism and the incorporation of iron into hemoglobin. Throughout his long scientific career he focused on only one disease, polycythemia rubra vera, the true abnormal increase of red blood cells.

He became one of the world's foremost experts of this rather rare disease, and he was the founder and chairman of the National Polycythemia Study Group.

While waiting for plasma to defrost one day, I was talking with Julia, the chief technician of the blood bank. She was a good-looking woman and an excellent pianist, and she told me that she was going to marry LRW during the first week in March. It was Wasserman's second marriage, and the happy couple left on a honeymoon.

In fourteen months, I had earned a total of $1,462.50 and, of that, had saved $1,100. The rest I had spent on personal items, an occasional movie, and one baseball game. It was enough money to bring Nienke and my son over from Holland. I found two furnished rooms, a kitchen, and a bathroom on West 87th Street, a block and a half from Central Park. It was three flights up, the furniture wasn't much, and the neighborhood was poor. For two hundred dollars I bought a car from one of the medical residents at Beth-El, a Studebaker. In my inexperienced eyes, it appeared to be in good shape, and my American colleague, whom I knew well as a fellow medical student in Amsterdam, assured me that there was nothing wrong with the engine. He took me for the sucker that I was.

It was a long wait on the pier in Hoboken on March 10, 1957. Debarkation from the Maasdam went by class, and Nienke, whose trip was paid for by the Dutch government, had made the crossing in the ship's bowels. There they were; my heart jumped. The many months of loneliness fell away and I experienced a deep feeling of happiness. That lovely, familiar face, the shy laugh, the tears, and the embrace said it all.

"Well, here is your son," she said, and she pushed a little boy toward me. "Say hello to your daddy."

Frank took one look at the stranger and started to cry. He didn't want anything to do with me, didn't let me touch him, and for the rest of the day he hid behind Nienke's skirt. It was understandable, but it made me feel pretty lousy. Huddled in a little group, we waited that rainy day on the rapidly emptying pier for a customs officer. There wasn't much to inspect: clothes, toiletry, a few toys, and a box.

"What's in the box?" he asked.

"An antique Friesian clock."

"Open it."

How do you open a sturdy, nailed down wooden box on an empty pier? That man easily could have let us go, but no, he decided to take his time and wait.

Wait for me to find a dockworker with a crowbar who charged me five dollars to open the box. On 87th Street, we made it, the three flights, with the box.

"Oh, how nice. We can sit outside," exclaimed Nienke when she saw the fifteen by twenty feet of black-tarred roof in the back. However, that roof was not made with sitting in mind. For someone used to living in a house with a park in front and a garden in the back, our apartment must have been a big letdown for Nienke, but never, ever, no matter where we lived, did she say a negative word. She was always joyful and positive. Lucky me. Those first years weren't easy for her, and a lesser woman might have taken the next boat back to Holland. Not Nienke, the trouper.

Our second honeymoon lasted three days. We explored the neighborhood, found some shops nearby, and strolled through Central Park. Summer arrived early that year. We had no air-conditioning, and Nienke spent as much time as possible with Frank in the shade under the trees in nearby Central Park.

When Dr. Wasserman came back from his honeymoon, he started morning rounds as usual, by looking at the slides of the new patients, while we presented the patient's history and the physical findings. He and I were looking through our microscopes, with a countertop between us. Residents and fellows sat or stood around waiting for LRW to give his opinion about the slides, which could take quite a while. He lifted his head from his scope and looked at me across the counter.

"Who the hell gave you permission to take days off?" he asked in his raspy voice.

I looked at him and replied, "I hope you too had a pleasant second honeymoon."

The other fellows jerked to attention. Nobody, but nobody talked like that to Wasserman. For a minute, he looked as if he was going to eat me alive, but then, slowly, a grin formed over his face. He turned to the others and couldn't resist saying, "Why the hell don't you people ever say something like that?"

One night soon thereafter, I was called to the emergency room. The patient, a seventeen-year-old boy, was a transfer from Roosevelt Hospital, where they tried to obtain a bone marrow sample from the sternum, the breastbone. An intern was pressing a towel on the chest of the patient when I came in. Another blood-drenched towel lay on the floor.

"Let me have a look," I said.

The intern removed the towel and immediately blood seeped from the small hole where the doctor from Roosevelt had inserted the marrow needle. The patient's blood count showed severe anemia, a few bizarre white blood cells, and hardly any blood platelets. I tried to take a marrow sample, but didn't think that I had obtained any bone spicules, the small pieces of marrow from which we could make a smear on a glass slide.

"Don't use a towel," I told the intern. "Just press with your thumb on the hole and give it five minutes."

In the laboratory, my suspicion was confirmed; there were no spicules. At rounds the next morning I presented the patient to Wasserman. He looked at the few pathetic slides I had managed to make and blasted away.

"These are the goddamndest, lousiest slides I have ever seen."

"That's all I could get."

"Well damn it, why the hell didn't you get another sample?"

"I did," and I handed him another slide.

It had one tiny spicule, but that was just enough to make the dreadful diagnosis of acute promyelocytic leukemia, the worst type. The patient died the next day.

Beth-El was a big letdown after my three months in Sinai. Snapper offered me a residency with the promise that I would become chief resident after a year, but I turned the offer down.

"Thank you sir, but I cannot accept it."

He leaned back, his right elbow on the armrest and chin in hand.

"I'm curious to know why."

"Well, there are a couple of reasons. Sinai spoiled me, and this place can't come close to it. You are the only top-notch teacher here and…"

"Thanks for the compliment," he interrupted.

"Sinai is loaded with good teachers and the constant interchange with the other residents is something we don't have here."

"I agree with you. You mentioned a couple of reasons."

"I don't want to sound insulting, but Beth-El is too Jewish for me. It is a completely different culture and atmosphere from what I am used to, and I can never be part of it. Jews have an entirely different sense of humor that I frequently cannot appreciate. You know that I have never been invited into any of their homes? That would be unheard of in Holland. It's different in Mount Sinai. The doctors are friendlier, warmer, and worldlier than those here in Brooklyn. My wife and I are not big-city people; we need some space and better surroundings for our children. So, ultimately, we'll move to a smaller town."

Snapper stood up, walked around his desk, and put a hand on my shoulder.

"I appreciate your frankness, and I must say that I agree with you, especially the difference between the people in Holland and here. You realize of course that you can't just walk into a hospital like Sinai and ask for a job. So where are you going?"

"I don't know yet sir, but I'll find something."

"I'm sure you will. Good luck."

I saw him for the last time six years later. Beth-El Hospital had let him go, and he was down to a one-room laboratory in a VA Hospital. I had inherited his love for multiple myeloma and had written two articles about a new treatment of this fatal disease. He of course had read them.

"I want to show you something," he said.

He set me down behind his microscope and there was a single cell, a plasma cell.

"Don't you think that's a myeloma cell?"

It put me on the spot. There was no way one could make that diagnosis from looking at one cell, but I wasn't about to tell him that.

"Yes sir, I think you're right," I said, and he was pleased.

When I left he gave me a copy of his book *Meditations on Medicine and Medical Education.* The inscription read: "To Dr. Bartholomeus Hoogstraten with best wishes and kindest greetings from his old compatriot." It was signed I. Snapper.

5

GRASSLAND: THE TUBERCULOSIS HOSPITAL

"We can't go on like this," I said when I came home after the talk with Snapper.

"Don't you get a raise in July?" Nienke asked.

"Only twenty-five bucks, not enough to live on. I have no future at Beth-El."

"Why not?"

"It's not a good hospital. It is in a predominately Jewish neighborhood, and the patients will prefer to see a Jewish doctor, not me, and there is zero science in that place. It's not for me. We didn't come to America to be stuck in Brooklyn."

"Did you talk it over with doctor Snapper? You know he brought you here."

"Yes, I did, and he agreed with me."

I looked around, but there were not many opportunities available for me. I was still an immigrant with no proven value. As a last resort, I accepted a residency in the Department of Chest Diseases in Grasslands Hospital, Valhalla, New York State. It was actually a tuberculosis hospital, and the salary of a resident physician was augmented with so-called danger money of fifty dollars a month. This brought it to a total of $ 215 a month, which for us seemed a mighty sum.

One Sunday in June, we drove to Westchester to find a place to live, but we never made it. The Studebaker had trouble going up the slightest incline, and, when we reached a long gentle slope, the engine couldn't produce enough power for the car to keep moving. Nienke and Frank got out and walked ahead, while I nursed the lighter car ever so slowly forward. The exhaust produced huge black clouds, and Frank loved it. He called it a choo-choo train.

The next morning, I cornered the resident who had sold me the lemon for two hundred dollars, but he refused to give me back my money. Fortunately the hospital administrator overheard our heated conversation. He called me into his office and helped me buy a reliable secondhand Ford from his brother, who was a used car dealer. The four hundred dollars meant a fortune to us at the time, and Frank didn't like the car because it wasn't a choo-choo train.

I went to register in Grassland and a kindly lady, Mrs. King, helped me.

"Your monthly salary will be $215, but $21.50 will be deducted as a contribution to your pension fund."

"That doesn't leave me with much, does it?" I remarked.

"And your taxes will also be taken out of it. Let's see…that comes to take-home pay of about $178 a month. Can I have your address please?"

"We don't have one," I replied. "We really didn't have time to look."

"Well, maybe I can help. We have a big house."

For sixty dollars a month she rented us two rooms and a small alcove, which Nienke and I converted into a kitchen, without running water and no gas. We had $118 a month to live on. The rambling white house on Hunters Lane in Elmsford had only one bathroom for Mr. and Mrs. King, their grown son, and our little family. It worked, except that when the son finished taking his shower there was little hot water left, and you could cut the steam in the bathroom with a knife.

Work at Grasslands was a dull routine after the hustle and bustle of Mount Sinai and Beth-El. I missed the intellectual stimulus of a Snapper and a Wasserman. The director of the Chest Service, Doctor Childress, and several members of the permanent staff were former tuberculosis patients. He was a kindly man who ran a calm service. I never saw him angry, and his only way of expressing disapproval was a slight pursing of the lips.

Two-thirds of the patients on my forty-bed floor had active tuberculosis, and the other third were bums in transit; people who at one time had TB and had the scars to prove it. Nearly all were alcoholics and, despite a strict rule against alcohol consumption on the premises, they managed to get soused frequently. They migrated like the birds. They arrived at Grasslands in the spring, stayed during the summer months, and left in late September to find their favorite TB hospital in the warmer south. They were always welcome visitors in both places, because it kept the census up and that meant continued state funding. County hospitals, not unlike VA hospitals, do almost anything to keep their beds occupied, including keeping patients for excessively long times.

Two patients from that year at Grasslands stand out in my mind. Mr. S. was a forty-year-old successful salesman of Russian descent who, during long sales trips, spent his evenings in smoke-filled bars. He had a small cavity in his right lung, and his sputum proved positive for TB. This meant confinement in the hospital for four to five months, and he took it hard.

"Why me doctor? Tell me, why me? My disease is bad isn't it?"

No matter how hard his lovely wife tried to lift his spirits, Mr. S. worked himself into a depression. I took him to the X-ray reading room one day and showed him the pictures of two really bad cases.

"Look at the size of the cavities in this one. They are monstrous. Moreover, this patient has only half a chest. As a last resort, they removed his entire left lung and collapsed his ribs."

"My God, can I become like that?" he asked.

I put his X-ray up, but covered the name. He looked at it and couldn't find the cavity.

"Is this a normal chest?"

"No it isn't. This is your X-ray." I pointed to the small cavity. Mr. S. shook his head.

"Oh boy. I'm ashamed of myself," he said. "Here I am complaining and look at it. I really am one of the lucky people."

From then on he was a model patient and went around helping the other patients. It sped up his recovery, and after three and a half months he returned home to start a new career.

The second patient is burned forever into my mind by his last words. He was one of few patients who did not have TB, and he was not my patient. He had a perfectly round shadow in his right upper lung field the size of a golf ball. His sputum was negative for TB, and the staff unanimously agreed that he had a tumor, maybe even a benign one. Surgery was clearly indicated, but his resident physician could not persuade him to have the operation, nor could the attending staff, not even Dr. Childress.

"I'll never have an operation," he persisted.

The more we thought about this patient, the more he became a challenge. Here was the one person who could be saved, even if the shadow turned out to be malignant, because it was so early. One evening I went to his bedside, and we talked about his family, his job, baseball, and just things in general. I left after thirty minutes without mentioning his lung. Two days later I passed his bed.

"Hi Jerry," I said and walked on.

He called me back: "Doctor, you have a moment?"

"Sure."

"I know you all told me that it is a simple operation, and I accept that. But I know that it is going to kill me. I am not going to survive it." He shook his head as he talked.

I should have let it go right there and then. In Indonesia, we ran into a similar situation when a soldier had a premonition of death. The evening before he was scheduled to go on patrol he talked to his lieutenant.

"Can I be excused from patrol tomorrow sir?"

"Why?"

"This may sound strange, Lieutenant, but I'm not going to make it."

"What do you mean you are not going to make it, Wiebe?"

"I know I'm going to be killed sir. I know it as sure as I stand here."

"I can't give you that permission Wiebe, because then anybody can come to me with the same excuse. Look, it's going to be a quiet little patrol, and we'll keep a sharp eye out for trouble."

Every thing went fine the next morning, until a single shot rang out half a mile from camp, and Wiebe fell dead with a bullet through his brain. His buddy gave his lieutenant a farewell letter he had written to his family. He asked them to pray for him and added an admonition to his younger brother, "I'll be in heaven when you read this. You are now the oldest son. Help Mom and Dad and be good to them."

In the officer's mess that night the young lieutenant cried. "Oh God, I should have listened to him. How was I to know that this would happen? He was so calm when he talked to me, and he didn't plead at all. Why didn't his roommates tell me about the letter sooner?"

It took the lieutenant a long time to get over it, and now I had failed to pay more attention to Jerry's premonition.

"Jerry, it looks like a benign tumor, but it will grow and eventually become so big that you'll have to have an operation anyway. Only then, the surgery will be more complicated. There is also a small chance that it is a malignant tumor, a cancer. In any case, it'll kill you if you don't do something about it."

"What do you want me to do?"

"If it was my lung, I would have the tumor removed, but it is your decision."

The next day Jerry made up his mind, and three days later he had the surgery. It turned out to be a benign adenoma. He came back from surgery, but instead of being happy he was depressed and didn't speak a word. On the fourth post-operative day, his right lung collapsed, and blood accumulated inside his chest. He had to go back for another operation. On the way to surgery he passed me in the hallway and stopped the stretcher. He looked at me with angry eyes and spit out, "You, you did it. You killed me." He died on the operating table, and I felt miserable. However, I had no guilt feeling. I didn't do the surgery.

"Hello, is this Barth?"

I immediately recognized the raspy voice as that of Dr. Louis R. Wasserman. "I'd like to talk to you. Can you meet me in my office this coming Saturday, say eleven?"

I sure could.

"What do you think he wants?" Nienke wondered when I told her of the call that evening.

"How do I know? Maybe he wants to offer me a job."

That Saturday, I drove to 100th Street and Madison Avenue. For an important man, Dr. Wasserman had a very small office. It was barely large enough for a desk, a low couch along the left wall as you came in, his chair, and one chair for a visitor. Open shelves along the walls were loaded with books from floor to ceiling, not arranged in any specific order, not even by disease. Only he knew exactly where every book was.

On the wall facing the door he had left enough space for a large modern painting of flaming reds. Nobody knew what it represented. Several expensive artifacts were hidden in nooks and crannies. I later learned that he was a well-known collector of modern art. Visitors to his apartment were often amazed to see an urn by Picasso on the grand piano in his apartment.

"That's what I want Julia to put my ashes in," he liked to joke.

Chagall's "Lovers in the Garden" on the bathroom wall shocked some people. However, his proudest possession was foot-high doll dressed like a doctor in a white coat. It had a bone marrow needle stuck deep into the heart and a small plaque at the bottom that read "Dr. Louis R. Wasserman, from his fellows."

Four visitors could fit in that small office, two on the couch, one on the chair, but the fourth one had to bring in his or her own chair. The two on the couch had to get up very carefully; otherwise they would bump their heads against the shelves above. The desk was covered with papers, and manuscripts lay spread out all over the floor, some covered with a thick layer of dust. Wasserman was a stickler for perfectly spoken and written English, and he insisted on proofreading every manuscript written by the people in his department. Unfortunately he often took his time, to the chagrin and agony of the inpatient authors.

"Look here," he said after I sat down. "The National Cancer Institute has just started a new program of chemotherapy for patients with acute leukemia. They have formed a cooperative group to study patients by protocols, and we will become members of the Acute Leukemia Group B. I'd like you to help me manage that program here in Sinai."

He went on to explain some of the details, but I had already made up my mind. Here was a golden opportunity to work in one of the finest hospitals in the world. Moreover, it was a foot in the door of one of the most exciting new programs ever started by the NCI.

"You don't have to convince me sir, I'll take it," I said.

"Don't you want to know how much the job pays?" He grinned.

"Not really. I'm sure you'll be fair," I replied.

"Will four thousand do for a start?"

Will it do? It was a bloody fortune. We talked some more, and then he asked me a strange question.

"How much do you think you ultimately want to make in a year?"

I didn't know what to say. Heck, I was still new in the country and had no idea how much a doctor made at that time, let alone what he would make in the future.

"If I ever make fifteen thousand, I'll be happy."

He grinned.

"Well, my career is on the way," I said to Nienke when I came home.

"Did Dr. Wasserman offer you a job?"

"Yes he did, in a brand new program supported by the National Cancer Institute. I am to manage the program for Wasserman."

In bed that night it hit me. Why did he pick me? I only had three months on his service; he had four fellows, two third-year senior fellows, and a staff. I had a green card that let me into the country, spoke with an accent, had five years of military experience, and was years older than the other fellows. Maybe that was the reason.

When I told Mr. S. in Grasslands Hospital about it, he too was enthusiastic.

"You'll need an apartment closer to the city," he said. "Maybe my wife can help; she is handy in those things."

Nienke had just given birth to our daughter, Evelien, and I was too busy to look for a place, so we gladly accepted the offer. Three weeks later Mrs. S. called. "I found something in Yonkers that you may like. I'll pick you up this afternoon, and we can have a look at it."

It was a second-floor apartment of a three-story house on 584 Warburton Avenue. It comprised a kitchen, living room, two bedrooms, a bathroom, and a small room that could serve as a study. However, it was the view that sold us. Across the road were Lyons Park, then the Hudson River (where we could see ships go by), and the Palisades decorated the far bank of the river. Catty-corner from the house were a grade school, a kindergarten, and the fire department. In the back was a good-sized garden, which was bordered by the high wall of the New York City aqueduct. In addition, we had a garage. Who cared that we had to climb three flights of stairs to reach the front door? This place was ideal for us, and, to top it all off, the rent was reasonable. When I left Grassland, the county kept my contribution to the pension fund.

Father Milligan of Grassland Hospital wanted to return to Central Africa where he had worked as a missionary. He showed me photographs of his old mission and knew the name of every native nurse and assistant. "I would love to go back to the Belgian Congo, but the doctor says that my kidneys aren't good enough."

He showed me the report of his urinalysis, and there was some protein in his urine.

"What do you think?"

"I think you should go."

"But my doctor said that I should stay here where I can get the best treatment."

"That is true, but he cannot give you happiness, and it may be many years before it becomes serious. In the meantime you'll be with your African friends, doing what you really want to do with your priesthood instead of pining away at this dull job."

He decided to go. "I wish I knew what I should do with my furniture."

"I'll buy it from you," I said.

We were moving to the apartment in Yonkers and had no furniture.

"I'll give it to you."

"No, you don't. Even a poor priest can use some money when he travels."

We agreed on two hundred dollars and were both happy. The furniture had belonged to his mother; it was old-fashioned, strong, and in excellent condition. However, there was one problem: the bed. His mother, and later he, only needed a one-person bed. Nienke slept in it, and I used a mattress on the floor. It was a lousy arrangement, but it was the only one we could afford.

6

THE MOUNT SINAI HOSPITAL AT THE PARK

July 1, 1958, was my first day as a hematology fellow in Mount Sinai. In addition to the two senior fellows and four assistant fellows, there were two medical residents on three-month rotations. Without a doubt, this was one of the largest hematology services in the country, and it was still growing. A large number of hemophilia patients lived in the city and in Westchester County, and since Dr. Martin Rosenthal was the medical advisor of the National Hemophilia Foundation, we were always busy taking care of these unfortunate patients. There were at least fifteen leukemia patients in the hospital at any given time, and that figure was most often closer to thirty. Even for a relatively rare disease such as pernicious anemia we had a clinic twice a week. All patients, both private and non-private, were considered educational material and, when the list of the patients in the hospital was handed out during our weekly grand rounds, the count was usually sixty or more.

Lou Wasserman was recognized as the builder of hematology at Mount Sinai, but Dr. Nathan Rosenthal was the father. In the 1930s, he and his first fellow, Dr. Peter Vogel, worked out of two small rooms on ward H that he had converted into laboratories. He had invented his famous Rosenthal needle to aspirate marrow from the sternum. The aspirate was put in a sterile glass tube, which contained a little heparin to prevent the marrow from clotting while the doctor continued his rounds. In the laboratory, he smeared the marrow on glass slides, stained them, and looked at the cells under the microscope.

One day in the mid 1930s, Nathan Rosenthal received a telephone call from Dr. Hargrave at the Mayo Clinic. He wanted to come down to discuss something strange he had seen on the bone marrow slides of a few patients. The next week, Hargrave flew from Rochester, Minnesota, to New York City just to discuss a couple of slides. He showed Drs. Rosenthal and Vogel white blood cells that contained a peculiar, ill-defined, bluish gray material in the cytoplasm. This was of no great surprise to Rosenthal and Vogel, who had observed the same phenomenon in Mount Sinai. However, the question was why these cells had that stuff in them and what was the meaning of it? Was it an artifact or was it real? The three men did not come to a conclusion, and a disappointed Hargrave flew back to Rochester the next day.

Now the true detective work started in both hospitals, and Hargrave found the solution to the riddle first. He looked at the records of the patients with that strange bone marrow, and lo and behold, they all had the same diagnosis: lupus. That looked like more than a coincidence to him, and he immediately put the question to one of the patients.

"I have noticed something abnormal in some of your bone marrow cells, and in that of other patients with lupus. It may be nothing, but, on the other hand, it could be important. Would you mind if I did another marrow on you."

"Well, I don't like it, but if you can learn from it, go ahead doctor."

It doesn't take long for an experienced hematologist to obtain marrow, a minute or two. We first put the glass slides on the edge of the bedside table with about a half-inch sticking over the edge so that it was easy to grab them. Next we drew a small amount of procaine, a local anesthetic, into a syringe and attached a fine needle to it. We placed some sponges, alcohol and iodine solutions, and the Rosenthal needle on a sterile towel, and we were ready. Like most of my colleagues, I aspirated the marrow from the sternum. While maintaining a light conversation with the patient, we cleaned the skin of the aspiration site and injected a little procaine in the skin and on the bone. This was far less painful than when a dentist injects one's jaw. A minute later, the marrow needle was inserted through the skin, pushed to the bone, and, with a few twists of the wrist, forced through the bone. We knew we were in the marrow when there was a sudden give of the needle. We attached a larger syringe to the needle and then I used to say, "You'll feel this for one second." The patient nearly always answered and during the answer, I pulled the plunger up. We needed only little marrow, and it was all over. We quickly put a sponge on the aspiration site, took a hand of the patient, and said, "Here, press on it." While the patient pressed, we smeared the marrow on the slides, put a band-aid on the sternum, and thanked the patient. There was no nurse involved, no fuss, and most patients remarked that it had been much less painful than they had feared. Speed and the notion that there was nothing to it were especially important for the leukemia patients, because they frequently had to undergo several marrow aspirations.

Doctor Hargrave's patient was nevertheless a brave woman when she volunteered. One can only imagine how he felt when he didn't find the strange material in her white blood cells. Had he made a mistake the first time or had he done something different in the preparation of the slides? He turned those questions over and over in his mind, went through every step of the procedure, and couldn't find an answer. A few days later, he even called the patient.

"Can you think of anything that I did different this time?" he asked.

"No," she replied. "The only thing I can think of is that this time you did it in your laboratory. The first time you did it when I was a patient in the hospital. Remember?"

A light went on in Hargrave's brain. He then remembered that the patients had been in their hospital beds all the other times. This meant that the marrow had been in the heparin, in the tube, and in his warm breast pocket while he went around seeing the rest of the patients. An hour or so later, he returned to the laboratory to make the slides and maybe, just maybe, that time interval was important. It was indeed. When he obtained the marrow in his laboratory and put the tubes in a bath with warm water for an hour before making the slides, the material showed itself in the cells, and it was only seen in the marrow of patients with lupus. That hour was what he usually needed to complete his rounds. The famous lupus cell was born. It was not even necessary to look at the bone marrow, because the same phenomenon occurred in the white cells of blood taken from a vein in the arm, as long as the blood was in an incubator for an hour. One can imagine the enthusiasm with which Dr. Hargrave made his next call to New York. It had all been pure serendipity.

That is one of the beauties of medicine. With long hours and diligent detective work, the solution to a problem can often be found in the strangest corners.

In my opinion, there are four essential attributes for a successful career in any science.

Good brains are a given. I was fortunate in meeting Nobel Prize winners like E. Donnall Thomas, George H. Hitchings, Gertrude B. Elion, Rosalyn Yalow, and Peyton Rous, as well as scientists like William Castle, Gordon Zubrod, Jim Holland, Donald Pinkel, Bill Dameshek, Max Wintrobe, Jean Bernard in Paris, Jan Waldenstrom in Stockholm, Louis Wasserman, and Tom Frei. They all matched their vast reservoirs of knowledge with superb teaching. They came up with good ideas, followed these up with well-designed experiments and studies, and during the course of that work were able to create additional ideas. I put my brain a step or two below theirs.

Willingness to work hard is a second attribute. During my three-month rotation in Mount Sinai, I made the time to review the hospital charts of well over two hundred patients with multiple myeloma, analyzed the data, and presented the findings during Grand Rounds. That may have been one of the reasons why Wasserman gave me the job in the first place. I left our apartment in Yonkers at five o'clock in the morning and didn't return until late at night. Wasserman had given me an extra job, a paying job. Morning rounds started at eight o'clock, and, before that, I drew the blood on every private hematology patient in the hospital and from all patients who had suffered a heart attack—about 120 patients total.

I drew the blood by the light that filtered in from the semi-dark corridor. Without waking the patients, I felt for the bulging of a vein or a decreased resistance where the vein runs deep below the skin and inserted the needle. Nearly all patients with a heart attack were treated with coumadin to prevent further blood clotting, which required daily testing of their blood for the next thirty or forty days. When I came to the bed of a new patient, he or she would wake up and invariably switch the bed light on.

"What are you doing? What's going on?" was the normal reaction.

"I am going to take some blood from your arm. Now please put the light out, it blinds me."

After the first couple of days most patients slept right through the procedure. This blood drawing business paid fifty hard-earned dollars a month. At the end of the day, I made evening rounds with Wasserman on his private patients, and we rarely finished before 8:30 PM. Our children were long asleep when I came home, and I ate alone, often falling asleep in front of the TV set. Nienke really was the one who took care of our children, because I never had time to be much of a father to them. I knew what hard work was.

Luck helps enormously, and I was lucky during most of my career. I was lucky in 1953 when Snapper gave his talk in Amsterdam. In 1958, Mount Sinai was the right place to be when the cooperative group program of the National Cancer Institute (NCI) started. Luck was again with me when I decided to leave Sinai and was elected chairman of a cooperative group. Luck is very important.

Serendipity is the fourth important attribute. The word was coined around 1754 by Horace Walpole in "*The Three Princes of Serendip,*" a fairy tale of three princes who always made discoveries by accident and by using sound judgment. Webster defines serendipity as "*an aptitude for making desirable discoveries by accident.*" A prime example is the discovery of the stethoscope by a brilliant French physician, Renee Laennec (1781–1826). He got the idea when he noticed two children tapping messages to each other from opposite sides of a wooden fence. Before his discovery, doctors had put their ear on chests and abdomens.

A more recent example of serendipity was the discovery of the hereditary deficiency of C3 protein. A house staff physician in the Boston Children's Hospital examined a young boy who failed to thrive. He thought that it might have something to do with a low-functioning thyroid and drew blood to determine the level of an iodine component T3, but the messenger delivered the specimen to the wrong laboratory, the immunology lab. The technician probably thought that the doctor had made a mistake when he wrote the order, and she tested the blood for C3 instead. The level turned out to be very low, and the young doctor asked the mother for a blood sample. She too had a low C3 and so, thanks to a mistake by the messenger, the lab technician who decided that the doctor had made an error, and to a doctor who was smart enough to test the mother, a new disorder, hereditary C3 deficiency, was discovered.

I believe that having good brains, working hard, being lucky, and serendipity go hand in hand. A single discovery is often the most that a scientist can expect to make during an entire career. As a matter of fact, most true scientists have no idea how their scientific discoveries are made. Nobel laureate Sir Peter Medawar, in his treatise *Induction and Intuition in Scientific Thought,* said, "They don't know."

I never qualified as having experienced serendipity, but I came close in a minor way during my fourth month in Sinai. On October 17, 1958, the Blood Bank called me because the technicians had trouble typing the blood of Mr. V., one of my patients with acute leukemia. His red cells were type O, so he should have had anti-A and anti-B in his serum, but he didn't have anti-A. We gave him five units of type O blood without trouble and studied the blood and saliva of his wife, two children, and brother. All four proved to have normal type A_1 blood cells.

Dick Rosenfield and I designated Mr. V's red cells as type A_g and from then on, it became a simple matter of carefully watching his blood. He went into a complete remission that lasted until June 1959, and his cells remained type A_g during that entire period. Leukemia cells reappeared in his blood in June, and suddenly his red cells changed to regular A_1 cells so that he could now receive type A blood.

"Do you know your blood type?" I asked him.

"I am type A," he replied.

"Are you sure?"

"Oh yes, I am. I have something to show you," and he produced an identity card of the German army that showed him to be type A in 1944.

"But you're Hungarian and a Jew. How did you get into the German army?"

"I was in a concentration camp and was given a choice between going to the Russian front or dying in the camp."

The Germans had a desperate shortage of manpower in 1944, and few people know that they conscripted Poles from German POW camps to serve as cannon fodder. They used them especially in Southern France, where they quickly surrendered after token resistance to the American VI Corps that had landed on the beaches of Nice, Saint-Tropez, and Cannes. This was the first time I learned that they had even conscripted Jews to serve as sacrificial lambs on the front lines, and I wondered why they bothered to type their blood, because surely they would not give their own blood to a wounded Jew.

"Mr. V., why did they type your blood?"

"Doctor, you must understand. It was not so that we could have blood transfusions. They did it because it was regulation."

Thanks to this 1944 identity card, we had discovered that the leukemia could interfere with the expression of the A substance on the surface of red blood cells. There were few top blood bankers in the world at that time. Drs. Alex Weiner and Richard Rosenfield were the giants in New York City; in the Netherlands Jochem van Lochem was a leading figure in Europe, and in England Drs. Race and Sanger wrote "Blood Groups in Man," which for thirty years was the bible for blood transfusion specialists. News of our exceptional patient spread fast in this small world, long before we published the paper. Within months I received a telephone call from the University of Pennsylvania and was offered an all-expenses-paid trip to Tokyo to present my findings at the meeting of International Society of Blood Banking that was held every fourth year. Australian-born Ruth Sanger singled me out after my presentation, and we discussed the implications of our finding. She made me feel like a king.

In addition to these four factors, it does not hurt to possess the art of babbling, a word I recently learned on the golf course. We were waiting on the fourth tee, and my partner was busy talking with the other players in our foursome.

"You enjoy talking, don't you?" I asked.

"Oh, you mean babbling," he said. "We Americans love to babble, just talking about all sorts of things. Filling the time."

However, I think that there is more to it than just filling time. It is called networking, it expands the circle of contacts, and that can come in handy. My friend Dr. John Ultmann was the champion babbler of all oncologists and hematologists. John made a career by writing lengthy, authoritative review articles, and he became an internationally recognized expert in lymphoma. He was also the tower of strength behind the University of Chicago Cancer Research Center. During annual meetings, babbler John could be seen sitting sideways on a chair at poolside, fully dressed or with his jacket neatly folded at his side. His audience was dressed in swim shorts and sunglasses, and John did the talking, without sunglasses. An hour or two later, John would still be at poolside talking away to someone else. In wintertime, the hotel hallways or lounge took the place of the pool. John, who was elected the 18th president of the American Society of Clinical Oncology, died of the disease to which he contributed so much, lymphoma.

Perhaps I should have added babbling to my list of essentials, but I never knew how.

7

BECOMING A HEMATOLOGIST

Although Wasserman had selected me to run Mount Sinai's participation in the Acute Leukemia Group B (ALGB), I still had to become a hematologist. The Hematology Department was squeezed into an area about seventy by fifty feet in size at the far end of the third floor of the Berg Laboratory building. It consisted of a tiny office for the director, an area for the fellows to study the bone marrow and blood smears, the main lab in which five technicians performed the blood tests for the hematology patients and three good-sized research laboratories. Routine hematology was done on the second floor, and for his iron studies Wasserman had a separate laboratory on the first floor.

For the Saturday morning sessions, we selected the most interesting new patients for presentation to Dr. Wasserman. At eight o'clock sharp he began looking at the slides, while the fellows presented the history, symptoms, and physical findings of their patients. This lasted about an hour, and then we went to the wards to see the patients. Unlike Snapper, who like a general always walked in front, Wasserman walked somewhere in a group of ten to fifteen fellows. He excelled as a teacher, and he had superb bedside manner—a little rough maybe, but he sure had a way of putting a patient at ease.

As the senior fellow, I joined him for evening rounds on his private patients, and then he was really at his best, especially with the ladies. When we walked into the room of an anxious new patient for the first time, he usually ignored the patient, walked straight to the bedside table, examined the contents of the inevitable box of chocolates and said something like "Lousy chocolates" or "Don't you have better chocolates?" The patient never expected something like that, and it always relaxed them.

"What kind do you like, doctor?" and the next day there was another box, from which he never took a sample. His rapport with longtime patients was beautiful, light, and easygoing. One of his favorite patients was an old, emaciated woman with an enormous liver and spleen, and a hugely distended abdomen.

"How are you doing?" he asked while palpating her abdomen.

"Not so good. It's becoming awfully difficult to get a good gigolo."

He grinned, "Can't you ask one of your friends to lend you one?"

"Are you kidding, she would never get him back," and she laughed.

When it came to treatment, all kidding was put aside. His patients received the best and most intensive therapy, which enhanced his reputation as a superb hematologist. Patients came from all over the world, even from the Arab countries. We were not surprised when, during the war between Egypt and Israel, the Egyptian military attaché insisted on being admitted to Mount Sinai, a Jewish hospital, when he fell sick. He knew what was good for him.

During weekends, the fellows treated the hemophiliacs, completed the workup of new patients, and performed the daily specialty tests. However, most of their time was spent with the management of the yellow babies. In 1922, Professor Karl Landsteiner, the discoverer of the four main blood groups, joined the staff of the Rockefeller Institute of Medical Research where, together with Alexander Wiener, he discovered the Rh factor in the blood of the Rhesus monkey, a macaque monkey indigenous to India and China. When a woman is Rh-negative and her husband Rh-positive there is a fifty-fifty chance that the baby will be Rh-positive. The mother doesn't want to have anything to do with those unfamiliar red cells of the baby and starts to form an antibody against the Rh. If, in a subsequent pregnancy, the baby again has Rh-positive cells, the mother's body recognizes them as the enemy and responds by making a lot of Rh antibody, which finds its way through the placenta into the baby, where it begins to destroy its red cells. That process is called *erythroblastosis foetalis*. The baby becomes severely anemic and jaundiced, which can lead to brain damage. The mother also becomes deathly ill and may die, unless the pregnancy is terminated.

The hematology fellow went to the delivery room when Rh incompatibility was expected, ready to collect blood from the umbilical cord, race to the laboratory, and test the plasma for bilirubin. Levels approaching 20 mg% signified severe jaundice and that the baby needed an immediate exchange transfusion, replacing its own blood with compatible blood. For private patients the fellow assisted the attending hematologist; for ward patients the fellow did all the work. However, that was not the end of it. At three- or four-hour intervals, the fellow repeated the bilirubin test because during the first few days of its life the infant continues to destroy its own newly formed red cells. Then a second, and sometimes even a third exchange transfusion becomes necessary. One weekend I was involved with the exchanges of four babies, and when Monday morning rounds began, I was dead on my feet. It was all part of becoming a hematologist.

Every patient is a potential research project. The idea of being one may turn some people off, but in Sinai nearly all patients were more than willing to participate in research, as long as it was fully explained to them. On March 3, 1962, a thirty-three-year-old Puerto Rican woman was admitted to Ward H. She had delivered four children, the last one on January 11, and her diet had consisted of bread, pinto beans, rice, some cheese, and occasionally a piece of meat, but no vegetables. The normal hemoglobin level ranges between 12 to 15 Grams %, but during the last delivery in another hospital her hemoglobin was only 6.1, and she had been discharged with it. She had never attended a prenatal clinic, had not taken any vitamins or iron, and she had lost twelve pounds in the preceding five weeks.

The hemoglobin on this admission was extremely low at 2.6, and I suspected a pure folic acid deficiency as the cause. Most interesting to me were her very low white blood cell (WBC) and platelet counts. She was also depressed, forgetful, sullen, and did not talk with the other patients. Her hair was dull, and she had small ulcerations in the corners of her mouth. I gave her two units of blood to relieve her immediate symptoms, and then I was faced with a dilemma. The literature on folic acid deficiency always emphasized the anemia, but I wondered about the white cells and the platelets, and about her symptoms. What was more important, the anemia or the many other manifestations? What would be the sequence of recovery if I gave her folic acid?

I decided to seek answers to those questions, but did not tell the patient. She received all vitamins except folic acid and a folic-acid-poor diet of twenty-five hundred calories. Her platelet count remained low, the WBC dropped further, the hemoglobin dropped 1.9 Gm% from the transfused level, and she lost an additional six pounds. Phase II of the investigation began on day twelve, when I started her on 50 micrograms of synthetic folic acid daily, a tiny dose. Her neighbors in the other beds were the first to notice a change. The patient talked as if she had some catching up to do, and she even smiled. She became conscious of her hair, and the ulcerations healed quickly. She began to gain weight. Her platelet and WBC counts started to rise on the second day and reached normal levels of three hundred thousand and twelve thousand, respectively, on the twelfth day. However, there were no new red cells in her blood, and a repeat bone marrow still showed evidence of a marked folic acid deficiency. With the help of a nurse as interpreter, I explained what I had done.

"Tell her that I want to learn from her illness, and that she will be fine."

The nurse took a long time to explain what we had done so far, and the patient replied in an equally long-winded manner. I just sat there and smiled at her a few times.

"She said it's OK. She is happy if you can learn something," said my interpreter.

The patient interrupted her emphatically.

"She says that if other patients can learn from her, you go ahead. She is happy, no trouble."

The patient and I smiled, and I felt a lot better. What a beautiful woman.

On first day of Phase III she received five milligrams of synthetic folic acid and started a regular diet. The WBC count shot up to twenty-five thousand, which is about three times the norm. It was as if the bone marrow wanted to repay a debt long overdue. In addition, for the first time, we saw new red cells, and, four days later, twenty-six percent of her red cells were new ones. She gained another seven pounds and was ready to go home. A grateful patient and an even more grateful doctor thanked each other.

A conventionally large dose of folic acid would have masked the sequence of recovery. By using the micro dose, we learned that the brain was more important than blood. The patient's body decided what was most important in her emergency state, not the doctor.

We published our findings and left it to others to answer the many questions raised by our patient. Since this study took place, stringent rules and regulations have been put in place to protect the interests of the patient. In 1972, ten years after our patient, she would immediately have received large doses of vitamins and iron, and we wouldn't have learned a thing. However, that does not justify the fact that I had failed to ask her permission to do the study.

After 1960, our number of hematology fellows increased dramatically and ultimately peaked at seventeen; Wasserman had a ball. At quarter to six in the morning he picked up his briefcase with the initials LRW on it and walked the two blocks between his apartment on 1200 Fifth Avenue and the hospital. His first stop was the cafeteria where I usually met him and where he inevitably had a huge piece of watermelon. Dr. Hans Popper, another early bird, frequently joined us. After a quick visit to his sickest patients, he worked in his office until eight o'clock, when he was ready to meet with the fellows. The most memorable year was when Phil Lieberman, Louis R. Weintraub, Janet Cuttner, Nat Wish, Art Figur, Ilana Tatarsky from Israel, and Roberto Sanchez from Mexico were the more senior fellows.

Weintraub was one of the favorites. Like Wasserman, he was small in stature, smart as a whip, and he had a superb sense of humor. One day he showed up with a new briefcase, the exact duplicate of the one Wasserman carried, and in golden letters were the initials LRW. He carefully timed his entry into the lobby and, while waiting for the elevator, positioned himself next to Wasserman. Both men had their briefcase in hand.

"Good morning, sir."

Wasserman acknowledged him with a nod. Then his eyes fell on the briefcase, and his lips moved ever so slightly into a smirk.

"Nice briefcase."

"Thank you sir, I kind of like yours, too."

They *both* grinned. Weintraub later became a professor of medicine in Boston.

Phil Lieberman was a jolly, round-faced bachelor who moved from one fellowship to another. He and Weintraub formed a good pair. Phil had one weakness; he knew something about everything in medicine, and he always had an opinion, even when he didn't have personal experience. When one of the patients was diagnosed with tuberculosis, Wasserman looked around, "Well, how are we going to treat her?"

I was about to say something, but Phil beat me to it.

"In New York Hospital we gave them...," and he went on to describe the treatment, which in my opinion was old-fashioned, to say the least.

"All right, let's do it," Wasserman agreed.

"Now just wait a minute," I interrupted. "Phil, how many TB patients have you yourself actually treated?"

"Well, none myself," he admitted lamely, "But we did have two patients on our floor."

"And that makes you an expert? Your treatment hasn't been used in years."

Wasserman now remembered my residency in chest diseases. "What do you recommend, Barth?" he asked sheepishly.

"I recommend that we transfer the patient to the Infectious Disease Service where she will receive up-to-date therapy."

The patient was transferred. Actually, Phil wasn't an aggressive person; he was a really nice guy, and he went on to become an outstanding pathologist at Memorial Sloan-Kettering Hospital.

Janet Cuttner was my favorite, and she stuck it out with Wasserman the longest. She was always in a good mood. People who didn't know her better sometimes tended to take advantage of her, and then Janet could come out of her corner like a Scottish terrier, fierce, eyes blazing, and dress the person down in no uncertain terms. Janet became especially adept at treating patients with acute leukemia, so much so that when the great William Dameshek went on vacation he turned the care of his patients over to her. Janet achieved such outstanding results that even Jim Holland, the chairman of the newly established Department of Neoplastic Diseases, listened to her. She is an excellent teacher, and the numerous hematologists who completed a fellowship are uniformly grateful to her. I have never heard anybody say anything negative about Janet. She is a dear friend.

Ilana Tatarsky was a tough sabra and smart, like all fellows, otherwise they would not be at Sinai in the first place. She did not volunteer her opinion often, but when she did the others quickly learned not to argue too much. She had studied at the Sorbonne and had a charming French accent. She went on to become the director of hematology at the Rambam Hospital in Tel Aviv. Nat Wish and Art Figur were both quiet and hard-working, and it is no surprise that they had successful careers in private practice.

Roberto initially had a hard time keeping up with the other fellows because his foundation was not nearly as good. However, he worked very hard, spent long hours in the library, and listened. His brain was like a sponge, and he soon caught up. At his farewell party Ilana said to him, "Wetback, go home," and he laughed the loudest.

My "big" salary didn't stretch very far with a second baby to feed and a third on the way. Any chance to make some extra money was welcome. The first opportunity came in the form of blood transfusions. Before I went on night call one day, the senior fellow told me about a young girl with aplastic anemia who needed frequent blood transfusions because her bone marrow no longer produced cells. "Her father gave me fifty bucks last night because the transfusion went so well," he smiled.

The girl had one look at me when I entered the room to start the transfusion and began to cry. "Daddy, I want the doctor we had last night."

"I understand dear; let me talk to the doctor."

The father explained that the transfusion the night before went faster than any of the previous ones, and his daughter had been delighted. That gave me an idea; if the senior fellow had made the girl happy, I could do it too.

"If I promise you to do it just as fast as the other doctor did, will you let me do it?"

"No, you can't," she cried through her tears.

"Yes I can. I can even find the smallest veins in babies."

"Honey, this doctor is real good. If he says he can do it, then he can. Why don't you let him try it?" the father urged.

I wondered how many times the poor man had gone through this. Moreover, where was the mother? He continued talking and stroking the girl and finally convinced her. I went back to the nursing station.

"Were you on last night?" I asked the nurse.

"Yes I was."

"Do you remember what needle the doctor used for that transfusion?"

"I think it was a twenty gauge," she replied.

"Give me an eighteen."

That blood ran in so smoothly that it took fifteen minutes less than the night before, and a grateful dad gave me seventy-five dollars.

That same month I had to start a transfusion in a man who was high up in the ranks on Wall Street. It was seven in the evening, and for once, I planned to go home early.

"Doctor, would you mind sitting with me while the blood runs in?" he asked—no—he begged.

There is not much you can do when a patient asks you for something like that. He talked about his family, his work, and his travels. He talked. The man was obviously very nervous about the transfusion. When it was finished, and I had the needle out, he thanked me and gave me fifty dollars.

"You look tired," Wasserman said one day, "You sleeping well?"

"No sir, not really."

I never called him by his first name. It was always sir or Dr. Wasserman, the European way. The other fellows and the residents called him Lou, but I couldn't, even though I was senior to the others. I was absolutely flabbergasted one day on rounds when, with all the fellows present, Gabe Jenkins, the senior medical resident of ward H, came over and out of the blue said, "You know, Lou, you're full of shit," and Wasserman only grinned.

I explained the bed situation to him.

"Do you have anything to sell?" he asked.

"I have a Leitz monocular microscope," I said.

We used only binocular scopes in the laboratory, and my scope was no longer of much use to me. It did have superior lenses though.

"I'll give you two hundred dollars for it, and you can buy a bed."

Back in the laboratory, we mounted a camera on the scope, and for several years I used it to take photographs of slides. My old scope, at one time the pride of my family, had found another home.

8

COW #8 IS DEAD

We were not quite sure why Nick Leone joined us for a three-month fellowship in 1960. Perhaps, after several years working as a dentist, he had looked in enough mouths and switched to medicine. He and I were older than the other fellows were. He had friends in many places, and his charming wife was the only female admiral in the U.S. Navy. He was interested in the effects of fluoride in man and animal and mentioned that when he finished his three months with us, he would go to Logan, Utah, where the Department of Veterinary Science of Utah State University had maintained a herd of cows on four different diets of fluoride for eight years.

The farmers in Northern Utah had long complained that the nearby Bethlehem Steel plant poisoned their cattle. The plant used fluoride for its steel production, and some of that fluoride not only contaminated the water but also spread over the land via the factory's smokestacks. The farmers claimed that the fluoride not only reduced the milk production of their cows but also caused them to lose weight and become less fertile. Bethlehem Steel listened to their claims and donated funds to the veterinary school to study the problem. In April 1952, a herd of thirty-two Holstein-Friesian calves was divided into four groups and for eight years each group was fed a different daily diet of fluoride: ten, twenty-five, fifty, and hundred parts per million (ppm). The cows were slated to be slaughtered in order to study the long-term effects of fluoride on every organ. I jumped.

"Why don't you and I study their blood before they kill them?"

Nick thought it a great idea and so did Wasserman. We called the plant manager and explained what we wanted to do. He agreed to fund our trip to Utah. I flew to Salt Lake City where Nick met me at six o'clock in the morning at my hotel. On our way to Logan City, we had breakfast at a restaurant famous for the largest and best-tasting steaks. Dr. LeGrande Shupe, chair of the Department of Veterinary Sciences, and his staff waited for us when we arrived at Science Station. A huge man of Swedish descent, "Tiny," as he was known, immediately tried to pull a fast one on me.

"Fluoride really did a piece of work on these animals." He grabbed a cow by its head and pulled the mouth open. "Look at it, the poor animal has no front teeth left in its lower jaw."

I was born and raised on a farm and knew all about cow's teeth. "You show me a cow with lower front teeth and you've got a miracle on your hands."

"Well I'll be darned; I thought you were a city boy," Tiny said with a laugh. "You gentlemen must be tired and hungry."

"No we are not. We are ready to go to work if you are," Nick replied.

We were determined not to let these vets get the best of us.

One by one, twenty-nine cows were led into a shed to be bled. Three animals in the hundred-ppm group had died in the interim years from infection, which statistically speaking was more than a coincidence. Drawing the blood from a cow was ridiculously easy. A worker led the animal into a stall, pushed its head through a frame, and when Tiny pulled the cow's head a bit to the side a huge, inch-thick vein popped up. "Don't be afraid if you spill a little," he joked. "This cow's got plenty."

Other vets joined our little group, including the retired chairman. Everything went fine until it was the turn of cow #8 to donate blood. She was a little skittish, and a vet had to push her from behind so that Tiny could get a hold of her head. He bent the neck, and I stuck the needle in. That is when #8 rolled her eyes and went to her knees.

"Get up, you dumb cow." The vet behind her gave her a kick, but #8 did not budge.

"We better revive her," said Tiny. "Barth, you massage her heart and, Nick, you pull her tail."

"Massage her heart? How am I going to do that?"

"Jump on her chest man, that'll do the trick."

I climbed on top of the cow, put my arms on the sides of the stall, and jumped up and down. In the meantime, Nick pulled her tail. Number #8 didn't move.

"That cow is dead," volunteered the retired chairman.

"Stimulate her anal sphincter, Nick. Perhaps that'll revive her," LeGrande Shupe encouraged.

Nick carefully put a finger in #8's ass.

"Not a finger, you dummy; use your fist."

That suggestion was too much for gentleman Nick. He looked up at the faces of six grinning vets, and we knew we had been had. Cow #8 remained deader than a doornail.

Unfortunately, our bone marrow needles turned out to be useless because the bones of the fifty- and hundred-ppm cows were as hard as a rock. On the morning of our last day, we walked past a large hall and saw a strange sight. From a tackle in the middle of the hall hung a cow by one of its hind legs. The blood of the dead animal drained from a cut in its neck into a bucket held by one of the professors.

"What are you doing?" I asked.

"I'm trying to measure the blood volume of a cow," he replied.

"Like that?"

"Not a good idea, eh?" he said rather sheepishly.

"Not really. You need isotope-labeled blood if you want to be accurate."

The professor got up from the floor, looked at the mess he had made, and shook his head. "That was a dumb thing to try," he mumbled and left.

I flew back to New York with my blood samples safely stored in special containers normally used to transport bull sperm. That is precious stuff, and the airline handled it carefully. The results of our many tests were interesting. When the fifty- and hundred-ppm animals were combined, their blood contained less gamma globulin, iron, and folic acid than the blood of the other animals. There were no differences in blood counts or in the functions of the thyroid and the liver. Of course, the three deaths in the hundred-ppm group were highly significant, and the farmers won their claim.

We reported our findings in the *Journal of the American Medical Association* where they drew the attention of public health officials. The Irish government invited Nick and I to testify on fluoridation of drinking water, but I could not leave New York, so Nick went alone.

I then wanted to study the effect of fluoride in the patients with multiple myeloma, a disease often accompanied by severe loss of calcium in the skeleton. The chairman of medicine would not hear of it. During a cocktail party a few months later, I discussed the idea with Dr. Frank Gardner from Boston, and, three years later, he reported extensive recalcification in a patient with advanced myeloma at the Federation Meetings in Atlantic City. A few old fuddy-duddy professors immediately attacked him.

"Didn't Dr. Gardner know that fluoride was bad for the teeth?"

I spoke up in support of the study, adding that fluoride mainly affected developing teeth, not those of patients with terminal cancer. Cohen and Gardner published their results in a 1964 issue of the NEJM and in 1966 in the JAMA. Subsequently, two large cooperative groups studied 150 patients with myeloma. The cows had provided a stimulus.

9

LEUKEMIA: THE WINDOW TO CANCER RESEARCH

Because chemotherapy used to be the treatment of last resort for patients with cancer, it still has a bad reputation. However, chemotherapy means nothing more than the treatment of a disease with chemicals. It is as old as surgery and medicine in general. In his 1970 lecture to the American Society of Clinical Oncology, Sir Alexander Haddow of the Chester Beatty Research Institute in London reminded the audience that some forms of cancer chemotherapy were used for at least fifteen hundred years with such diverse agents as belladonna, antimony, aconite, mercury, and arsenic. He considered the therapeutic effects of these substances illusory, trivial, unproved, or at the most, fleeting. In 1767, Burrows best expressed the opinions of contemporary authors (*A New Practical Essay on Cancers, London*):

> ...whatever has been proposed for the curing of cancers, are merely palliative medicines; and that no real specific has been hitherto discovered for that fatal disorder, although the physicians of all nations, from the time of Hippocrates to the present have, by numberless researches and experiments, made trial of every thing in nature, from the most innocent drug, to the most virulent poison, both in the mineral and vegetable kingdoms; yet the disease still baffles the power of physic...

Nine years later, Peyrilhe flatly stated "every attempt to cure cancer, by any method which is to restore the diseased tissues to a healthy state, is not only vain but also absurd" (*Dissertation academique sur le cancer*, Paris, 1776). Burrows' opinion remains appropriate for the many forms of quackery that even in modern times continue to plague the public by self-serving, fortune-seeking so-called healers.

Of the many agents used in the Middle Ages and before, arsenic has continued to fascinate pharmacists and physicians. The Roman physician Aulus Cornelius Celsus (42 BC–37 AD) first mentioned it as a medicinal. In the 1700s, Thomas

Fowler developed a solution of arsenic trioxide in potassium bicarbonate and claimed it to be useful for a wide variety of diseases such as pemphigus, asthma, and chorea, also known as Saint Vitus's dance. The most famous use of arsenic was in the form of Salvarsan, introduced in 1909 by Dr. Paul Ehrlich as a cure for syphilis. Doctors used this until the mid 1940s when penicillin took over as a more effective and less toxic drug. Even then, arsenic refused to give up, and it has made a remarkable comeback.

In 1992, four Chinese physicians, Sun, Ma, Hu, and Zhang, reported in a little-known Chinese journal that they had successfully treated thirty-two patients with acute promyelocytic leukemia (APL) with a solution of arsenic trioxide (As_2O_3) and herbal extracts. Having long been the worst form of leukemia, APL patients usually died in days or weeks, but these authors claimed a much longer survival. Six years later, Drs. Zhang, Wang, and Hu reported excellent results with arsenic trioxide in seventy-two patients with APL. This remarkable result was confirmed in 1998 in a *New England Journal of Medicine* article by twelve authors from the Memorial Sloan-Kettering Cancer Center and the Cornell University Medical College in New York City. They treated twelve patients (one for each author?) and, with little magnanimity, made the following statement, "It is intriguing that we and the Shanghai investigators both found that virtually all patients with the confirmed diagnosis of APL attained remissions." In the next paragraph, they state with a touch of arrogance, "Although quite preliminary, our data suggests that arsenic trioxide is active in APL." Never mind that the Chinese investigators had given the New York doctors the idea to try it. A prestigious journal and scientists from a renowned institution could not find a way to admit that they had come in second.

Mustard gas, that infamous poison of the World War I, gave the impetus for modern cancer chemotherapy. In World War I, army doctors noticed a marked drop in the white cells and platelets in the blood of gassed victims. During the interval between the two world wars, scientists on both sides of the Atlantic Ocean wondered whether the gas could also inhibit the growth of experimental tumors in laboratory animals and some exploratory studies were underway when World War II broke out. Under the cloak of strict secrecy, scientists received permission to study nitrogen mustard, one of many types of liquid mustard.

In 1942, three pharmacologists at Yale University, Drs. Alfred Gilman, Louis S. Goodman, and Frederick S. Philips, received a contract from the Chemical Warfare Service to conduct basic investigations with nitrogen mustards. Four years later, they published a report about their biological actions and therapeutic applications. In 1963, Gilman recalled their experience.

> "There they were in early 1942 all set for the first experiment; Philips with a stopwatch in his one hand, paper and pen in the other, Goodman and Gilman with a battery of syringes on the table in front of them and a hoard of rabbits in cages ready to be injected. Their colleagues kidded them that the enemy surely had no intention to attack with hypodermic needles. The most important observation they found in the rabbits was a remarkable sensitivity of lymph nodes. The lymph cells in these nodes just seemed to disappear, leaving only skeleton tissue."

They convinced Dr. Thomas Dougherty in the Department of Anatomy to study the mustard in mice with experimental lymphoma. Dougherty had successfully transplanted lymphoma from one mouse to another, and he knew that after such transplantation all the animals died in about three weeks. It so happened that he had one mouse with a particularly large tumor. "We couldn't wait to get a whole group of animals, so we gave the mustard to this one lone mouse," he wrote. That lone mouse happened to respond and lived for eighty-four days. They subsequently gave the drug—for that is what they called it now—to many other animals, but never again achieved such a remarkable result. In most forms of mouse leukemia, they obtained no effect at all. Ten years later Dougherty said, "I have often thought that if we had by accident chosen one of these leukemias in which there was absolutely no therapeutic effect, we might possibly have dropped the whole project." One lone mouse made history, and, in retrospect, it was sheer serendipity."

Following this single encouraging result, Dr. Gustav E. Lindskog, a young assistant professor of surgery, agreed to try the mustard in a patient in the terminal stages of lymphoma. He had no idea what dose to use, and on advice from Goodman, gave 0.1 mg per kilogram body weight daily for ten days. Since the drug was still classified as top secret, the entry in the patient's chart read: *0.1 mg. per kg Compound X given intravenously.*

The result was dramatic. By the fourth day, the patient felt better, and on day ten the large tumor masses were no longer palpable. The white blood cell and platelet counts remained normal, and the doctors were elated; little did they anticipate what came next. The blood counts dropped precipitously and for the next couple of weeks hovered around zero. In the meantime, they made a serious error in judgment; they did not wait to see what would happen to the first patient and treated another patient with a ten-day course. The bone marrow of that second patient was wiped out for several weeks, and worse, the patient did not respond. From then on, they advised a more conservative dose, and nitrogen mustard ultimately became a very useful drug in the treatment of Hodgkin's disease.

These early experiments left a deep impression on the investigators, best exemplified by a letter from Dougherty to Gilman in 1962. In the last paragraph he wrote, "You might be interested that I still have practically all the blood films, bone marrow and the sections of the organs, etc. of both mice and men treated at that time. I have thrown out a few blood films, but could not bring myself to throw this part of my life completely in the ash can."

In 1954, a Congressional committee invited NCI officials and other expert witnesses for a hearing on cancer. The members of the Senate and the House form a close-knit community, and several of their wives had cancer or had already succumbed to the disease. Chemotherapy, a new treatment of cancer, became a magic word for these politicians, something they could take home to the voters. The Senate Appropriations Committee encouraged the NCI to start a "directed" program for leukemia similar to the wartime antimalaria program. To get the program off the ground the committee added one million dollars to the budget for fiscal year 1954. The NCI staff and its advisers shuddered at the thought of a scientific program controlled by congress and certainly didn't like the idea of limiting the program to leukemia. But a million dollars talk, and soon a few hastily formed ad hoc committees reached agreement on three points: The program would be developed on a basis of "voluntary" cooperation, would not be limited to leukemia, and would be directed by the NCI.

The National Institutes of Health opened a new Clinical Center in 1953, and Dr. Charles Gordon Zubrod became the first Clinical Director of the NCI. Gordon, as we all knew him, hid a very active mind and a zest for action behind a stoic exterior. He had never treated a cancer patient, but he was convinced of the ultimate success of chemotherapy and was therefore willing to devote his life and career to the new program. Little did he anticipate how much resistance he had to overcome. Dr. William Crosby of Walter Reed Army Hospital wrote that leukemia was incurable and that patients should only receive supportive therapy. Tufts University School of Medicine's Dr. William Dameshek, the editor of *The Journal of the American Society of Hematology*, condemned the mere thought of giving chemotherapy to these poor patients. Ten years later, he and I played a game of chess during the Federation Meetings in Atlantic City.

"Are you still trying to treat acute leukemia?" he asked.

"Yes I am."

"You better find something else of interest if you want to make a name for yourself. Leukemia is a dead end."

Dameshek was not only a poor chess player but he also could not foretell the future.

Tom Frey, in John Laszlo's 1996 book *The Cure of Childhood Leukemia*, mentions that when he presented a new combination chemotherapy program for acute leukemia during a 1963 meeting of the National Cancer Advisory Board, Dr. Carl Moore, the president of the International Society of Hematology (ISH) and a member of the board, commented that the presentation struck him as being outrageous. Moore, who never treated patients with acute leukemia, sent me a copy of his new book, thanking me for my work during the New York City meeting of the ISH. The frontispiece of the book consisted of the portrait of a young man with huge enlargement of the lymph nodes in his neck and the subtitle read *Hodgkin's Disease: A Uniformly Fatal Disease*. A few years later, Moore turned out to be dead wrong, because aggressive chemotherapy helped cure the disease.

Crosby, Dameshek and Moore wrote many editorials in which they condemned the use of chemotherapy in leukemia. Their pessimistic attitude had an enormous negative influence on the other members of the Advisory Board and the medical community at large. British oncologists met with similar skepticism from their peers. Sir Ronald Botley Scott, Physician to H.M. The Queen, said in his July 9, 1970, lecture before The Royal College of Physicians, "Surgery, radiotherapy and hormonal treatment still reign supreme." He never used the word *oncology* and no one dared mention chemotherapy around him. Despite such outright opposition and skepticism from their peers, a younger, more adventurous generation of hematologists plodded on against overwhelming odds.

Leukemia is by far the best disease to study the effects of chemotherapy. Solid tumors require repeated surgical biopsies to study the biology and progress of the cancer, but we could take a blood specimen every day if necessary. The first protocol study in which Mount Sinai participated compared methotrexate (MTX) with 6-mercaptopurine (6-MP) and with a combination of the two drugs.

"Why don't you ask doctor Hodes whether we can enter his children on the protocol," Wasserman said to me shortly after we entered our first patient. Hodes, the chairman of the Department of Pediatrics, was not exactly a friend of LRW, but his department did not have a staff hematologist, so there was a chance.

"Why me?" I asked.

"Because he doesn't know you," Wasserman grinned.

That afternoon I saw Dr. Hodes in his office.

"What has that to do with me?" he asked after I explained the new program.

"We would very much like to enter children with acute leukemia on the study and make Mount Sinai's participation in this National Program all-encompassing."

No matter what one said about Hodes, he always had the best for Sinai at heart.

"Why didn't your boss ask me?"

I responded with the faintest of smiles.

"You're not a second Louis Wasserman are you?" he grumbled.

"No sir, and neither am I my master's voice."

That drew a smile. He pointed a finger at me. "All right, but I want you to look after my children."

"Thank you, sir. I'll take good care of them."

On my way out, I thought how ridiculous it was. One department chairman delegates me to talk about an important program to another chairman. That man has never met me, he does not know that I am a newcomer to hematology, and yet he wants me to take charge of his little patients.

"He said OK," I reported back to Wasserman.

"Good." He grinned at the good news.

"But only if I take care of his patients."

The grin faded.

"And he doesn't want a second Louis Wasserman."

The grin was back.

Thus Mount Sinai became one of the few institutions to enter both adults and children in the studies of the ALGB and was soon one of its largest contributors. I will never forget when a technician showed me a tube with some blood of one of the first children. "What is that?" she asked. The bottom portion of the tube contained a red fluid and a larger top portion was whitish.

"That, if I am not mistaken, is a layer of white cells on top of the red cells."

Normal blood contains about one thousand red cells for every white cell. This child had 1.2 white cells per red cell. It was the worst presentation of acute leukemia I would ever encounter. The WBC dropped so fast after the first treatment that the kidneys could not keep up with it and the little girl had a temporary kidney shutdown.

The whole idea behind the study was based on our knowledge that leukemia cells multiply at a much faster rate than normal white blood cells do. Our two drugs, MTX and 6-MP, both interfere with the multiplication of cells, good ones as well as bad ones. If we could wipe out the leukemic cells before the drugs caused too much harm to the good cells in the bone marrow and the rest of the body, then maybe—just maybe—the marrow would recover by making only good cells. However, we walked a tightrope with every patient; when the doses of the drug were too high, the patient could die, and when the doses were too low, the leukemia thumbed its nose at us.

Initially, investigators from eight institutions entered patients in the ALGB study, and every four months we met to discuss its progress and to develop new studies. Wasserman and I flew to Washington together for our first meeting.

"Look, the people you are going to meet are big and very smart, and I want you to keep your mouth shut. I just want you to listen," he warned me.

"Yes, sir."

The meeting was held in a small conference room next to the animal quarters of the National Institute of Health. Around a single table sat about twenty participants, who didn't look big and didn't act big, but they were very smart. Tom Frei turned out to be a tall, skinny man with a friendly face and a balding head. He led the meeting with easygoing authority, while Jim Holland and J Freireich (he doesn't want a period behind the J) did most of the talking. The other members included G. Watson James III from the University of Virginia, Charles Spurr from Bowman Gray, Rose Ruth Ellison from Buffalo, Farid Haurani from Thomas Jefferson in Philadelphia, Ross McIntyre from Dartmouth, and Harvey Rothberg from Princeton.

Soon after the meeting started, it became clear that Freireich challenged Holland. He was loud, at times vulgar, sarcastic, and wild. By his own admission, he made a career of being an unpleasant person, a task at which he was eminently successful. Jim was the calm Princeton sophisticate who easily parried J's attacks. Frei was the arbiter, using tact and humor as well as profound knowledge. The other members hardly said a word. Then Frei mentioned that a new drug called Endoxan would soon be available for clinical testing. It came from the Asta Werke in Germany. Wasserman had already heard about it and had found a TWA pilot to bring him some of the drug. I used it in a few patients and apparently was the only person in the room with some experience with the drug.

"We gave it to some of our patients," I said.

All heads turned to me.

"Well, can you tell us something about it?" Tom asked.

I told them how we had experimented with the drug and had arrived at a safe dose, whereupon Tom asked me to chair the study of Endoxan, soon to be known as Cytoxan.

"I thought I told you to keep your mouth shut," Wasserman said on our way back.

"Yes, you did and look what it got us into when I said something."

The results of the MTX and 6-MP study were published in 1961. It was the largest study of its time and the first in which a combination was tried of two drugs that work in entirely different ways. We had hoped that the combination would lead to more remissions than either drug alone could, and it did. Unfortunately, the remissions did not last long and there was no improvement in survival. It was still only five months for children and about four months for adults. Only seven of 101 patients with acute myelocytic leukemia (AML) responded with a remission, and one of them was Mr. V., my patient who had the change in blood type.

Mr. V. was a model patient. His white blood cell count dropped to zero with the treatment, and the number of platelets was too low to count. I'll never forget when Claude Kaplan, one of our technicians, came into my office with a big smile. "I saw a few platelets in Mr. V."

When Claude said something like that, one had better believe her. Sure enough, the next day there were sufficient platelets for a count: four thousand. Normal is one hundred fifty thousand or more. However, it was enough to predict that Mr. V. would go into remission. At that point, he developed pneumonia, which he survived thanks to antibiotics and superb nursing care. After two months in the hospital, he was in a complete remission and went back to work. Eight months later the blue spots reappeared; he had relapsed. He stubbornly continued to work, staying on his feet for eight hours a day. He clung to life with tremendous willpower as long as he could and when it was his time to go, he went in complete peace, with a loving wife and children at his bedside. His last words to me were, "Thank you. I die a free man."

In 1960, I presented the initial results with Cytoxan to a panel of experts, and in 1962 we published the final results. There were only two complete remissions in adults, so that the drug was a complete failure, at least for acute leukemia. All patients died in a short time.

10

THE PIONEERS

Who were those physicians that treated this hopeless disease? How could they face the continual failures? Were they immune to the many deaths? What did their colleagues think of them and of their work? Did their failures have an effect on their family life?

In 1960, my third year in hematology, I gave a talk on the presentation and treatment of acute leukemia to the staff of the Department of Internal Medicine. Standing in the pit of the old surgical amphitheater, I looked up at the semi-circular rows of benches packed with white-robed men and women. Front and center sat the director of medicine, the great Dr. Alexander B. Gutman, flanked by the identical twins Drs. Richard and Mortimer Bader. Gutman was the founder and editor of the prestigious *American Journal of Medicine*, the so-called Green Journal. The fun-loving, heavyset Bader boys were his co-editors. They were impressive men indeed for a fledgling hematologist to face.

I finished my presentation by comparing the survival graphs of 1955 and 1960. The medium survival time for children had moved from 4.4 months to 4.5 and for adults from 3.9 to 3.6 months. In other words, there had been no improvement at all in those five years, and the outlook was still miserable. There was no applause when I finished the presentation, and nobody had a question; there was only dead silence. Finally, either Richard or Mortimer—I never could tell them apart—leaned forward.

"Let me ask you something, doctor," he said. "Since you have not seen any change, and they're all going to die anyway, why do you even treat these poor people?"

It was a question I hadn't anticipated, and it made me think for a moment.

"Because, doctor, you do not."

The amphitheater emptied while I gathered my slides. The Bader twin who had asked the question stayed behind. He slowly slid his bulk off the bench and came down to me in the pit.

"Hi, I'm Richard," he introduced himself. "That was a gutsy answer and a very good one." He thought for a moment and added, "You people must be a special breed to be able to stand losing your patients day after day. I certainly couldn't do it."

He had hit the nail on the head. We *were* a special breed, and, initially, there *were* very few of us. We were a rather disorderly bunch that tended to break the rules and create new ones. Our constant failures made us insecure in many ways and vulnerable to our own doubts. Not many hematology fellows selected a career in cancer research after exposure to acute leukemia during their first year of training. We were eternal optimists and never appeared depressed in front of a patient; instead, we were uplifting and full of empathy, warmth, and understanding. We gave until at the end of the day there was little left to give. Nienke recognized when the barrel was empty, when I needed warmth and loving to recharge my batteries. We were not robots and without the giving from our spouses, few of us would have made it. Our unflinching enthusiasm was sustained by our never-ending hope that we were on the right track, that there would be new drugs, better drugs, and that one day we too would see some of our patients survive. It was a hope that now and then was strengthened by a special patient such as Mr. V. Without that hope, we too would have been crushed by the numerous failures.

Some oncologists do not make it; they give up and escape to pathology, anesthesiology, or hospital administration where they do not have to face patients. Two of my friends changed over to psychiatry; another became a famous pathologist. When I started, we had in our armamentarium only six drugs, which had limited use in a few diseases. Nitrogen mustard was effective in Hodgkin's disease; busulfan and chlorambucil worked only in chronic leukemia; TEM was touted for a while but turned out to be of little use; that left MTX and 6-MP for acute leukemia. Chemotherapy for the so-called solid tumors such as lung and breast cancer came much later. In his presidential address to the American Association for Cancer Research of April 8, 1971, Jim Holland said of our difficult beginning, "The antileukemic drugs could be counted on one foot of a three-toed sloth, albeit slowly."

It was up to the hematologists to get chemotherapy off the ground. We treated our patients with acute leukemia and saw them die—all of them. We were not made of stone and, yes, we were affected by our constant failure. The deaths of some patients hurt more than that of others did, but we tried hard not to bring that hurt home with us. Moreover, if standing at the bedside of a dying patient were not enough, we also consoled the family and learned at times to be priest, minister, or rabbi.

Finally, some hope came in the form of a letter from Dr. Joseph Burchenal of Sloan-Kettering in New York City. In this 1963 letter to the members of the American and the International Societies of Hematology, Joe asked who had seen children with acute leukemia that had survived five years or longer.

"I don't know of any, do you?" Wasserman asked me.

"One, a little girl," I replied. Lou did not follow the children.

Joe's letter opened our eyes. Just asking whether we had seen any patient with acute leukemia survive five years was already remarkable. Could it really be true that we were achieving some minuscule success? Burchenal received the reports of 159 patients from around the world and with it, he established the Acute Leukemia Long-Term Survival Registry. He later reported an interesting statistic. Of the 159 documented cases, 24 died in the 6th year from the diagnosis of their disease, 12 in the 7th year and 11 in the 8th year. After eight years in remission, the likelihood of a relapse became very small, and ultimately sixty percent of these long-term survivors had not relapsed after nine years. Joe could now proclaim that there were cures in a disease that used to be uniformly fatal. What made these 159 cases so remarkable was that they had been treated with the only three drugs available, Methotrexate, 6-MP, and cortisone. As I was writing these lines, I looked up the membership directories of ASCO and ASH, and Joe was not a president of either. Neither organization honored this deserving scientist with a presidency.

Tom Frei called from the NCI one day. "Barth, we have a patient from New York City who wants to go home. We gave her a new drug, and she is ready to be discharged. Can you take over?"

"Sure Tom. Is there anything I should know about the drug?"

"It is a vinca alkaloid from Eli Lilly. We have given her one dose of vincristine."

I had never heard of vinca alkaloids. "How much did you give her?"

"Only 10 milligrams."

When the patient arrived in Sinai she was completely paralyzed, something Tom had forgotten to mention. She never recovered. It didn't take us long to learn that the 10-mg dose was at least five times too much, and even one milligram can cause unexpected trouble. Years later when vincristine, also known as oncovin, was a well-established anticancer drug, one of our patients, a barber, complained of pain in a small area of his right shoulder immediately after the injection of the 1-mg. The nurse did not think much of it and told him to rub his shoulder. When I saw him one week later, he could not lift his arm above the horizontal. The nerve in charge of lifting the arm was dead. This unique side effect remained a mystery and unfortunately, it happened to a barber who could no longer practice his livelihood.

Oncologists are often asked to explain what they mean by acceptable toxicity. The answer depends on the degree of success. If the drug gives only twenty percent responses in patients with advanced breast cancer, both patient and physician may decide that severe vomiting is not acceptable. However, if there are sixty percent long-lasting responses, most patients are willing to pay the price of that toxicity. Adriamycin causes a lot of vomiting and has several other side effects, but it is also a most active drug for advanced breast cancer. Therefore, the women are willing to endure the toxicity. Similarly, Cis-platinum causes severe vomiting, but it is very active in testicular cancer. Seven times Tour de France winner Lance Armstrong received both drugs for his cancer of the testis that had spread to his lungs and brain, and he is now a most-effective spokesman for cancer chemotherapy, despite the fact that he puked, felt miserable and lost all his hair. There is no need to ask him whether it was worth it.

Unfortunately, some investigators report extraordinarily good results with a new drug or combination of drugs without having sufficient data on which to base their conclusions. In the early 1960s, during the Federation meetings in Atlantic City, Dr. Freireich from the NCI claimed to have achieved complete remissions in eleven of thirteen adults with acute leukemia who were treated with a new agent with a very long name, methylbisguanylhydrazone. It was a huge breakthrough and too good to be true.

"From which dusty shelf did you pick that stuff," Jim Holland asked.

Freireich ignored the dig, and ALGB began a large study of this drug. We soon shortened its long name to methyl-GAG, because the patients vomited their guts out. In over ninety patients, we saw only two responses, which we considered nothing more than background noise.

"How do you account for that minor discrepancy, J?" Jim asked.

"You people don't know how to treat leukemia," J replied sarcastically.

Janet Cuttner from our lab was furious. "I'll take our way of treatment any day over yours," she fumed.

At the next ALGB meeting four months later, Freireich and group statistician Ed Gehan explained that if an agent produces no antitumor effect in fourteen consecutive patients with the same tumor type, that agent has a ninety-five percent chance of being ineffective for that tumor. Conversely, if it produces fourteen successive remissions, it will be a success in ninety-five percent of patients.

"We should have treated a fourteenth patient," Ed said lamely.

That was sheer nonsense, because they already claimed eleven remissions in thirteen patients, which we had never seen before. The NCI doctors could not duplicate their own result. Methyl-GAG went back to the dusty shelf and from then on, I was skeptical of all of Freireich's claims.

11

DR. CHARLES GORDON ZUBROD

Charles Gordon Zubrod was born on January 22, 1914, in Brooklyn, New York. In 1932, he entered the College of the Holy Cross and spent his summer vacations driving a Good Humor truck, averaging fifty dollars a week. His father was a partner in a brokerage firm and a member of the New York Stock Exchange, but the Depression was in full swing and he could barely keep his head above water. He certainly could not afford to send his son to college for the second year. Father Dolan, the President of Holy Cross, offered tuition and board to Gordon, who as a student waited on tables, worked in the library, and won a cash prize in chemistry. He graduated *magna cum laude* and went back to Good Humor to earn the money for medical school tuition. In 1947, Holy Cross sent him a bill for the tuition plus 6% interest.

In 1936, Gordon entered the College of Physicians and Surgeons of Columbia University in New York City. Again, he waited tables in the cafeteria and picked up free meals. He was also the night cashier for Good Humor in Baldwin, Long Island, an experience that helped him get the full-time summer job as cashier at Bard Hall, the medical school residence. There he met and fell in love with the credit manager's secretary, Kay Mullins. He called her Kaki, and they married on June 15, 1940.

After finishing medical school, Gordon worked for six months in a State Mental Hospital on Long Island while waiting for an internship to start at the Jersey City Medical Center. However, as he wrote in his book *Stairway of Surprise,* the Holy Spirit and Kay intervened and he began an internship in the Presbyterian Hospital instead. He tells a story about a patient with a bacterial infection of the heart. On March 6, 1942, Dr. Martin Dawson handed him a syringe with a brown liquid and said, "Zubrod, this syringe holds some of the penicillin I've made—$10,000 worth—and I want you to give it to this patient." It was just enough for one patient and Gordon gave the recommended course of 7,000 units every four hours. Unfortunately the patient died.

That story reminded me of my own experience when I lay wounded in an army hospital on Java in 1947. The Dutch army doctors had just received the first batch of penicillin, and I started on a course of forty injections, 7,000 units every three hours, not four. After the fortieth dose, my temperature was still elevated and I was condemned to another forty shots. The fever came down, but rose again after injection number seventy and after the next one.

"You think I may have become allergic to the stuff?" I asked the surgeon.

"I don't know. They didn't tell us anything about toxicity."

"Do you mind if we skip a dose?" I had visions about a third course if that fever persisted.

"No, fine with me. Let's see what happens," he agreed.

The fever stayed away and I was permanently allergic to penicillin.

During his residency in medicine, Gordon went to see Dr. James Shannon in the Goldwater Memorial Hospital on Roosevelt Island in the East River. Shannon conducted clinical and pharmacological trials in malaria for the war department. He invited Gordon to help him, and since he had to start his military duty anyway, Gordon joined him as a first lieutenant in the Army Medical Corps and had his first experience with controlled clinical trials. In 1954 Shannon, who had left Goldwater for the NIH, suggested that he apply for an opening at the NCI. He interviewed with the scientific director, Dr. Burroughs (Bo) Mider, who offered him the position as clinical director with a starting salary of fifteen thousand dollars. He was not board certified and had never treated a cancer patient. Immediately after his appointment, he called the chief resident of medicine at St. Louis University, Dr. Emil (Tom) Frei and offered him a job at the NCI. Tom treated cancer patients when they were admitted to the Department of Medicine, but he had no formal training in oncology for the simple reason that the medical schools did not yet offer such programs, and the word *oncology* did not even exist. Like the rest of us, he started from scratch.

At the NCI, Gordon met Jim Holland, who was interested in acute leukemia, and together they designed a trial comparing two regimens of methotrexate. When Jim left a month later for the Roswell Park Institute in Buffalo, they agreed to conduct the study in Bethesda and Buffalo. Gordon soon realized that it would take an inordinately long time to complete the study in just two institutions, and he invited other clinics to join them in the effort. It was the birth of the first cooperative group, the Acute Leukemia Group B (ALGB), with Tom Frei as the first chairman. Tom invited Wasserman to join the group and Lou asked me to run the program at Mount Sinai. We soon became one of the largest contributors.

In 1963, Tom Frei resigned as group chairman. He moved to the MD Anderson Cancer Institute in Houston and soon thereafter became chairman of the Southwest Cancer Chemotherapy Study Group, the SWCCSG. In a power struggle for the chairmanship of the ALGB, Jim Holland was the easy winner over J Freireich. He asked me to chair the multiple myeloma studies.

The fascinating history of multiple myeloma began when, on a warm day in August 1844, Thomas Alexander McBean vaulted from an underground cavern at his house near London. He felt something snap in his chest and was in agony. Doctor Thomas Watson put him in a plaster cast, told him to rest, and for good measure bled the poor man a few times. The pain receded, probably because his broken rib healed, but returned in the spring of 1845. A course of "steel and quinine" enabled him to travel to Scotland, where "he bounded over the hills as nimbly as his companions." Mr. McBean died on January 1, 1846, and his bones were studied by Dr. John Dalrymple, who reported his findings in the *Dublin Journal of Medicine* under the title *"Mollities et Fragilitas Ossium"* or "Soft and Fragile Bone." In 1989 von Rustizky, a Russian physician, described a patient with eight tumors in the bones and he gave the disease a new name: multiple myeloma. This is the disease of the plasma cells that fascinated Isidore Snapper so much.

A year before I took over the myeloma studies a few reports appeared in the European literature about a new drug called Melphalan. Danny Bergsagel in Houston, Elliot Osserman in the Presbyterian Hospital across town and I decided that each of us would study a different dose schedule. My first patient had such severe bone pain that the staff did not dare touch his bed.

"David, I am going to give you a new drug that I know little about."

"Anything doctor, anything to get rid of the pain."

"I'll try, but I can't promise that it'll help."

David closed his eyes in pain, "Please do it."

He received a loading dose of 10–12 milligrams (mg) per day for a week, and he actually became pain free. His blood counts dropped for three weeks, and when they recovered, I put him on a maintenance dose of 2–4 mg per day. I selected this schedule for the first ALGB study and two years later we reported the results in sixty-four patients from ten hospitals. Two-thirds of the patients had a good response, and our dose schedule is still recommended in the Physician's Desk Reference forty years later. In a second study, we repeated the same loading dose every five weeks, but without giving a maintenance dose. The result was less impressive, because in between courses the pain came back in too many patients. Danny and Elliot had similar satisfactory results, and myeloma had become a treatable disease.

In 1965, Jim asked me to become chairman of the Lymphoma Committee. I called Al Owens at Johns Hopkins, who chaired the lymphoma studies of the Eastern Cooperative Oncology Group.

"Al, how would you like to do a study together?"

"That'll be interesting, Barth. It'll certainly help patient recruitment."

"I have an idea about combining several drugs that I'd like to talk to you about."

"Fine with me, Barth, but let me first discuss it with Bruce."

Dr. Bruce Shnider of Georgetown University in Washington, D.C., the chairman of ECOG, agreed. A week later, I flew to Baltimore. Al, his associate Ray Lenhard, and I agreed to compare a low dose of Cytoxan with a high dose and with a combination of Cytoxan, Vincristine and Prednisone. This was the first combination chemotherapy study in lymphoma ever undertaken, and the results, published in 1968, showed superior remission rates for the combination. However, I will never forget what Dr. David Karnofsky asked, ever so quietly, when I finished presenting our results at a meeting of the National Lymphoma Task Force. "Dr. Hoogstraten, ultimately, what good did it do for the patients?" Ultimately meaning, did they live longer and was it quality living? I had no answer.

Next, Jim and I put our heads together and we decided on a daring new approach in the treatment of Hodgkin's disease, combining chemotherapy and radiation therapy. Again, I approached Al Owens, and, again he readily agreed to participate. I next called Gordon Zubrod. "Gordon, Al Owens and I would like to study combined chemotherapy and radiotherapy for Stage III Hodgkin's disease."

"Well, that's a new idea."

"So new that I haven't even discussed it with the radiotherapists. I first want to know whether you'd agree to let us do the study."

"I don't see why not, as long as it is well thought out."

"Thanks, but now comes the tricky part. I can't talk to the radiotherapists without offering a carrot. I'll need to promise them some financial support; otherwise they'll never do it."

"Barth, you mean that I have to give the money, right?"

"Right—it is only fair, because the chemotherapists are already supported."

"OK, if you can come up with a well-designed study, I will give financial support for the radiotherapy."

"How much, Gordon?"

"How much do you think you need per patient?"

"I figured eight hundred." I knew that was too much.

"Will you settle for six?"

Of course I would, but I had only cleared the first hurdle. The next one would be more difficult—how to convince the radiotherapists to participate and how to get them to agree on doses of radiation, on the fields to be radiated and on a schedule of radiation? Great Britain was the bedrock of radiotherapy in the 1950s and 1960s, and fortunately, Dr. Simon Kramer, the radiotherapist at Jefferson University Hospital in Philadelphia, was a Brit. We had never met.

"Yes Dr. Hoogstraten, what can I do for you?"

"Sir, I chair the lymphoma studies of the ALGB and I'd like…"

"Excuse me, what is 'ALGB?'" he interrupted.

His question showed how far apart we were. I explained ALGB to him.

"Al Owens and I propose to do a study on Hodgkin's that will include radiotherapy and I'd like to come to Philadelphia to discuss it with you."

"By all means do, if you think it may be worth your while."

Dr. Kramer was all for it after I explained some of the details.

"You realize of course that without some funding, the radiation therapists will not cooperate and the study will never get off the ground," he said after we had agreed on the design of the study.

"How does six hundred dollars per patient sound?"

"That will do the trick. That is very reasonable, as a matter of fact, but can you get it?"

"I am a step ahead of you. I had that guarantee before I came."

He liked that, and promised to send me the details on the radiation in two weeks.

When they arrived, I put the protocol together and sent copies to four prominent oncologists: Henry Kaplan and Saul Rosenberg at Stanford, Tom Frei in Houston, and Ralph Johnson at the NCI. Several of their suggestions and comments were included in the final draft of the study and we were now on solid ground. Simon and I arranged a meeting with the radiotherapists of the participating institutions to explain the study and answer their many questions. We wanted to radiate all the lymph nodes in the body, the so-called total nodal therapy. Only two therapists at the meeting knew what we were talking about and we had to teach the rest on the spot. Even well into the study, I continued to receive calls from hesitant therapists.

The results of the study exceeded our expectations. All patients treated with chemotherapy followed by total nodal radiation went into a complete remission (CR). In the group treated with total nodal followed by chemo, the CR rate was an amazing eighty-six percent. The survival of the patients in these two treatment arms was far superior to that of the other patients. We presented our data at the 1971 Symposium on Hodgkin's disease sponsored by the National Cancer Institute and published the end results in March 1973.

Zubrod established cooperative groups in different regions of the country. At one time there were no less than twenty-two groups, each with its own headquarter and statistical office. The Cancer Chemotherapy National Service Center (CCNSC) managed this massive enterprise at the NCI, and the group chairmen met a few times a year at the NCI to discuss problems and exchange information with Gordon and, later, with his successor, Dr. Vince DeVita. We formed a Chairmen's Committee and elected Jim Holland as our first chairperson. Two years later, I succeeded Jim.

We all regard Zubrod as the father of chemotherapy and the creator of NCI's cooperative group program. The program began in 1955 with an initial budget of five million dollars and three groups, Acute Leukemia Groups A and B and the Eastern Solid Tumor Group. In 2002, the program involved sixteen groups, more than fifteen hundred institutions and approximately twenty thousand new patients entered the cancer clinical trials of the groups that year. Thousands of individual physicians now participate and the Southwest Oncology Group has grown from about nine hundred members in March 1981, the year I resigned as group chairman, to 4,898 twenty years later.

Gordon retired from the NCI in June 1974 to become the director of the newly formed Miami Comprehensive Cancer Center and Nat Berlin joined him as Deputy Director in 1987, the year his wife Kay was diagnosed with Alzheimer's disease. Two years later Gordon retired to care for her. Nat introduced the Zubrods to the Wassermans and we were frequent visitors at Lou and Julia's Medridge Farm in Sandy Hook, Connecticut. Gordon, a born athlete, easily showed us up in water skiing on the nearby Housatonic River. I thought that he was a naturally shy man and was touched when he told me of being awkward in social gatherings. "I lacked the easy grace of classmates," he wrote in his book. "The lack of social finesse was a cloud on a bright horizon."

I know the feeling so well. During my high school vacations, I pushed a cart loaded with bricks and cement through the streets of Hilversum and saw my classmates go by in their tennis outfits. They had fun, laughed, and I hoped that they didn't recognize me. The feeling of awkwardness and trepidation has diminished over the years, but it has never quite left. It now pleases me to no end to see how natural our children are in social settings, how they use first names in company where I would use only last names. Gordon said that he was a loner—in a way, so am I.

In 1971, his peers honored Gordon with the presidency of the prestigious American Association for Cancer Research. When President Nixon signed the National Cancer Act, he gave Gordon one of the pens, which he promptly lost. Twenty-seven years later, his son found the pen and mounted it for his father's eighty-third birthday. It galls those of us who knew and admired him that he never received an award for his monumental work. He should have received the Nobel Prize or the General Motors Kettering Prize. In August 1997, he sent me a copy of his book *Stairway of Surprise*, which had just come out. He started it as an autobiography, but his children and granddaughter Crissie converted it into a family tribute to Kay, Gordon's wife of nearly fifty-eight years.

In 1998, he called me to say that Kay had died on April 11. In his May 14 letter, he wrote how the entire family had gathered the day before for her eighty-fourth birthday. He described in *Stairway of Surprise* how Kay and he had climbed the stairway of life together and how Kay always selected the right door to enter, saying, "Gordy, this is the one." When he asked how she knew, she replied, "It's easy; I just ask my Friend, the Holy Spirit." In my letter to him, I wrote, "Kay no longer needs to ask her Friend which door to open. She passed through her last door and took the extended hand of her Friend. I wonder—is this a sad or joyous happening?"

I sent Gordon the final computer printout of my book, *Eyes of the Blind*. "Once I started reading I couldn't put it down," he wrote and then was kind enough to correct some typos. Charles Gordon Zubrod died on Tuesday, January 19, 1999, at age eighty-four. He too passed through the final door.

12

TELLING THE PATIENT THE DIAGNOSIS

How does one tell a patient that he or she has cancer? How do you tell parents that their child has leukemia? Few medical schools give courses in bedside manners, and students and house staff officers can only learn from the example set by their elders. Few attending physicians and professors take the time to teach this long-neglected art. I have witnessed the blunt, matter of fact approach of some doctors and wondered why they had bothered to study medicine. Two episodes in particular come to mind.

The pathologist of Danbury Hospital in Connecticut and I were looking at the blood smear of a young boy when the family physician walked in. "What do you think it is?" he asked. It was acute lymphoblastic leukemia and as the hematology consultant for the hospital, I would probably be involved with the treatment of the two-year-old boy.

"You want me to tell the parents?" I asked.

"No, I'll do it, but come along and I'll introduce you."

In the corridor on the way to the boy's room, he mumbled to himself. The young couple waited anxiously.

"Johnny has leukemia," the doctor blurted out when we entered the room. Just like that, without any preparation, he gave the poor parents the worst possible news. The young father screamed like a wounded bull, the mother cried in her handkerchief. There was not a darn thing I could do at that moment. Why had that doctor been so insensitive? Later that day he stopped me in the hallway and asked whether we could talk. It was obvious that he was deeply troubled. "I love those people," he said. "As we walked to Johnny's room I was rehearsing how I was going to give them that terrible news. I was going to be so gentle with them, but then I blocked it all out and said the stupidest thing I could ever say. I blew it so badly and wanted to do it so well." The man was miserable and he carried that disastrous episode with him for the rest of his life. The parents asked me to take the care of their child.

"I can't do that. I work in New York City and come here only once a week. You still need a local doctor."

"I can't go back to that doctor," the father said, tightlipped. "No way."

"Yes you can," I said. "Do you know that I saw that man actually rehearse what he was going to say? He was going to be so kind and then botched it completely."

"But why didn't he let you tell us?" the mother asked.

"Probably because, being your doctor, he thought it was going to be easier for you if he did it. In other words, he tried to be very considerate. Why don't you give him another chance?"

They looked at each other.

"Would you mind if I give you some rather personal advice?" I asked.

"No, please do," replied the mother. She was apparently the stronger of the two.

"We'll treat Johnny and hopefully he will go into a remission, but beyond that I cannot give you much hope. You will go through a difficult time emotionally and I think that it will be much easier for both of you if you have another baby. Why don't you try while Johnny is still with you?"

They went back to their doctor; the boy did go into a remission and the mother did get pregnant. Three months later, tragedy struck twice; she had a spontaneous miscarriage and Johnny relapsed. I stuck my neck way out. "Get pregnant again, and I still will keep Johnny alive until you have the baby."

Fortunately, Vincristine had been recently introduced and, together with prednisone, Johnny went into a second remission. He subsequently relapsed and died three weeks after his mother delivered a baby girl. The lives of the parents could go on. They moved to another state and had three more children. For many years I received a Christmas card from them. Nienke put them on our Christmas tree.

The second episode took place that same year. One day Wasserman was particularly concerned about admitting an elderly woman with leukemia. Fifteen seconds before eight o'clock that morning, I began calling the admitting office and although I kept calling for five minutes, we didn't get a bed. Wasserman behaved like an angry tiger.

"Goddamn it, when are they going to build more beds? Jesus Christ, what a lousy way to run a hospital."

That afternoon I was writing a note in the nursing station on the sixth floor of the Klingenstein pavilion when a doctor walked in. He seemed upset.

"What's the matter?" I asked.

"Oh, I just had to tell a patient that he had prostate cancer and he took it very hard. I hate it when I have to do that."

I finished writing the note and went down one floor to see another patient. While we talked, a large shadow flashed by the window. I looked out and down below saw the body of a man draped over a fence; it was the patient with the newly diagnosed prostate cancer.

"What was that?" my patient asked.

"I don't know. A large bird, maybe. Will you excuse me a minute?"

I went to the nursing station and called Wasserman.

"A patient from room 656 just committed suicide."

"Thanks," Wasserman said. He immediately called the admitting office, and that evening his patient was admitted to room 656.

I can sympathize with doctors who find it difficult to tell patients and their loved ones of the diagnosis of a fatal disease in such a way that it reduces the pain. One should not expect every doctor to be capable of doing it. It is never easy, not even for those who have done it many times. A good bedside manner is the first step toward the alleviation of the anxiety that every patient experiences. It is the beginning of a warm interaction between patient and doctor. Patients are often reluctant to give information that may be important for the doctor to know. After the house staff failed to obtain a vital piece of information, it took an old-timer like Dr. Snapper to find out that the aforementioned Mr. Mullhead had an identical twin and that the twin had recently had an operation.

Students and house staff officers are lucky when one of their professors takes the time to discuss with them how he or she ought to tell a new patient about a bad diagnosis. This is how I advise them to handle it: "Take a chair or sit on the edge of the bed if need be and touch a hand. That will comfort the patient—and don't think for a minute that men do not appreciate that gesture; they do. Unless the patient decides differently, it is better when the spouse, a close member of the family or a good friend is present. Remember that it will be awfully lonely for the patient after you leave the room. Tell them the bad news, but immediately hold out a few rays of hope for them to grasp. Be prepared to answer the questions that will follow, not once, but several times, because most patients do not remember what you told them. You will be amazed how well-informed patients accept the worst diagnosis and how grateful they are that you took the time to sit with them. Answer all questions and remember: The informed patients become your best patients. No question is a dumb question."

Oncologists are sometimes surprised by the apparent ease with which patients accept their diagnosis. I was crossing the hallway one day when the desk clerk stopped me.

"Doctor Hoogstraten, can you help this man?"

The man appeared to be in his early twenties.

"What can I do for you?"

"I have leukemia," he said, just like that, and it momentarily stumped me.

"You, uh…have a doctor?"

"No, that's why I'm here. A doctor in Bloomsburg, Pennsylvania, did a blood count and he said that I had leukemia."

"Do you have the report with you?"

"No, I figured that I'd better see a doctor in New York."

A quick blood count and smear confirmed that he had chronic myelocytic leukemia and Janet Cuttner took him on as a patient. "He is the easiest patient I ever had," she said a few weeks later. That statement is true for the vast majority of cancer patients. They know that their oncologists are doing the best they can, that they are fighting for them. Although the treatment with radiation and chemotherapy causes side effects that range from discomfort to outright misery, they go through it with few complaints. They join the fight.

The women fight in their own quiet way. The men tend react differently. "Doc, I'm going to lick this. I'm going to fight this like hell." I have never heard, nor can I imagine, hearing a patient with a heart ailment saying those words. The word *cancer* does that to people; it is an enemy. They marshal their strength against that enemy and that brings out their inner beauty. Their resolve and beauty makes being an oncologist so gratifying.

During the era from 1950 to 1970, most hematologists did not tell their patients that they had leukemia, Wasserman among them. "You have a rare form of anemia, but we'll take care of it," he usually said. At that time the word *cancer* was rarely used in front of a patient. Only relatives were told, outside the room, usually in the corridor.

"What did the doctor tell you?" the patient invariably asked, and then it was up to the relatives to talk around the "bad" word. Patients often avoid mentioning that they have cancer. Men especially will frequently say only that they have "The big C," or some other euphemism. When chemotherapy began to show some better results and give added hope to patients and relatives in the 1970s, cancer—both the word and the disease—finally came out of the closet, so to speak. However, even today it remains subject to well meaning and sometimes misplaced sentiment.

"Doctor, we think it's better that you don't tell Dad that he has cancer," a son or daughter will not infrequently advise the doctor.

"Doctor, will *you* please tell Dad the diagnosis. It is better coming from you," another son or daughter of the same patient may say.

"No need to tell my family that I have cancer, doctor," the patient will say. Then, in the corridor, the family members will say, "Doctor, we know that Dad has cancer."

Three scenarios, and, if they are not careful, physicians can be caught in the middle. I always told my patients their diagnosis and the vast majority can take it, will calmly accept it. Many already sense it from the demeanor of the physician when he enters the room. As long as oncologists take their time to talk to patient and family there is no trouble in the telling and the acceptance of the diagnosis of cancer. *Time* is the operative word. A doctor who does not give that time is a poor physician.

It doesn't happen often, but sometimes a patient is uncomfortable with a doctor. Moreover, the reverse can also be true: The doctor may occasionally not be able to establish a rapport with a patient. When either situation occurs, it is best to not let it drag on, because both parties may feel it at the same time. Patients must feel free to ask for a referral to another physician and the physician should immediately recommend a qualified colleague. When a doctor is uncomfortable with a patient, he or she should speak up. It may even clear up a misunderstanding.

Of all medical specialists, I have the deepest admiration for the pediatric oncologists. They must not only deal with the parents, but also with children of all ages. The babies that cry when yet another needle probes for their tiny blood vessels. The four- and five-year-olds with whom the pediatrician can develop a rapport, a mutual trust. Wizened eight-year-olds with the bald heads who grasp the meaning and outcome of their disease; who move around from bed to bed while pushing their IV pole and talk with the younger children. The teenagers rebelling against their fate. Children may underestimate their parents, and some parents do the same with their children. At the end of a long day, the pediatricians are likely to be more emotionally drained than other physicians are and they are paid the least for their work.

Dr. Donald Pinkel, the first director of the world-famous St. Jude Children's Research Hospital in Memphis, Tennessee, expressed it best when he described his experience with the parents of his young patients. In John Laszlo's book *The Cure of Childhood Leukemia* he wrote, "The emotional and psychological impact was the same, no matter what the educational level of the parents. In fact, leukemia and cancer in general are great levelers. The highly educated and highly sophisticated people and those who are not sophisticated or well educated come to a common plane because it's something you have to deal with emotionally and not rationally. These sorts of things tear you up inside and your family and friends can't understand what's happening at times. Yet I'd rather face these problems and make progress for the children than not move ahead."

Don mentions how he too received advice not to pursue the work in childhood leukemia because "it's a dead end." Don, who only treated children, wrote about how, during the first five or ten years, he did not reduce the mortality. "There were many times when I left that ward in the evening and didn't know how I was going to retun to work again the next day. It could be devastating at times and I couldn't really discuss it with anyone, not even my wife. I knew that no one else could quite understand what I was going through." Don, your colleagues do.

A few years after Johnny, the boy in Danbury Hospital, died, I attended a most beautiful, deeply moving family affair. The patient was a twelve-year-old boy with advanced lymphoma. He no longer responded to radiation therapy or conventional chemotherapy and had volunteered for experimental drug treatment. He actually had to convince his parents to do it. A rabbi was Michael's most frequent visitor. He helped him prepare for his Bar Mitzvah. When he became just well enough to leave the hospital, I asked the rabbi when it would take place. I was not invited, but surprised the family by going to their synagogue in New Jersey and there was welcomed with open arms as Michael's doctor.

Women, children and men in the congregation wept openly when Michael read from the Torah, especially the Haftorah, the prophetic portion. He ended with a short sermon in which he reminded his family and friends that this was a joyous occasion and that they should be happy for him. Men and women pulled themselves together and the ceremony became the great festival it was meant to be. The highlight came when a member of the family, a well-known singer, gave a rendition of "Mack the Knife."

Michael died six weeks later, a man.

"Doctor, how long does he have to live?" "How long do I have?" "When is mother going to die? You can tell me, I can take it." "Doctor, you must tell me how long my father has to live." These are some of the frequent questions and statements oncologists will hear during their careers. Two weeks before I wrote this section, the topic of prognosis was discussed on National Public Radio. The moderator of the panel had invited a professor from Chicago who blasted physicians for not telling patients and relatives when the patient was going to die. "Doctors have an obligation to give patients and relatives a well-informed opinion about the prognosis. Patients have a right to know when they are going to die, but many physicians avoid giving answers. Loved ones also should know, because often they have to make the necessary arrangements. The doctor should deal with their concerns as well."

"Well said, professor," the moderator agreed.

"I was very angry because our doctor said that mother had six months to live and she died after only two months," said a hospice nurse. "He gave us false hope and he should have known better."

A second nurse was equally annoyed because the doctor had refused to say how long her father would live. "I pressed him and he finally gave Dad four months. But Dad lived for nearly a year and all that time we were in agony."

Not one of them had something good to say about doctors. "Lived in agony." It sounds so good, so dramatic, and so utterly nonsensical. That nurse should have been happy that her father lived so much longer. In addition, she should have known better than to press the doctor. The hospice nurse of all people had no business saying that the oncologist gave false hope. And that professor—if he was a professor—did not know what he was talking about. He too spoke of the agony of loved ones. Guests and moderators on such programs often include that overused "loved ones" phrase. Don't they realize how phony they sound? I have news for that professor: After forty years in the field I still cannot foretell the time of death; I can only give an estimate. Too often have I seen patients live far beyond the time I thought they would live, and, sadly, I have also seen them die sooner. Oncologists have learned to explain the outcome of the disease and not to give a definite time limit when it is impossible for it to be precise.

"In this form of cancer the prognosis varies anywhere from a few months to years. Let's see how you respond to the treatment first and then we'll have a better idea." That is one way to answer the question soon after the diagnosis is made. On the other hand, it is quite appropriate for a doctor to advise a patient to get his or her affairs in order. Why wait? It all depends on the rapport between doctor and the patient or a child's parents, not between a pushy relative and the doctor. After establishing a good rapport, the question of prognosis becomes a mutual understanding, a matter of trust.

"Doctor, am I dying?" or "Am I going to die?" Oncologists hear questions like these in their practice and they should not hesitate to reply positively. *The patient already knows.* The patient feels the need to talk about it when they pose the question; they need to be reassured that there will be no pain. That it will be peaceful. That is the time for physicians to be at their best, to make sure that the patient will not become isolated, that he or she will not be ignored. Unless the patient is asleep, the family must try not to discuss matters outside the door. Always remember that the patient is still part of the family. This is also the time when various support systems can be most helpful, such as the church or temple, community, school, and service organizations. In addition, please do not put on a somber face. It's all right to laugh with the patient. *Visitor, be yourself.*

Friends and family should speak freely and not hesitate to bring the latest news. Believe me, even those patients who know that they are going to die, want to know what is going on in the outside world. They are still part of this world and they demonstrated that very clearly in the following episode.

When Dr. William Dameshek reached the mandatory retirement age of 65 at Tufts, Dr. William H. Crosby succeeded him. I was in LRW's office when Crosby called and Lou put him on his speakerphone.

"Lou, Bill is driving me crazy. Either he has to go or I will go. Can you help me?"

"Barth is sitting across from me, Bill. Let me ask him." Lou turned to me. "Can you find a spot for him?"

In addition to being on the staff at Mount Sinai, I was the director of the hematology department at the Elmhurst City Hospital at that time. The New York City Department of Health had contracted with Mount Sinai to take over the medical care of this thousand-bed hospital.

"Well, I can use him to make rounds once a week, but I can't pay much."

"Did you hear that, Bill? Barth can give him an appointment. Let me talk to Bill tonight, and maybe we can work something out."

That is how the great Dameshek moved to New York City, and became one of my junior attendings. He had a tendency to talk down to the rest of the staff, but nobody could match his experience, and his anecdotes were both fascinating and informative. During one of his lectures in Mount Sinai, we learned that sometimes the patients are the best teachers. Dameshek walked on stage, stood behind the lectern and announced: "Instead of talking about the symptoms, diagnosis and treatment of acute leukemia, I like to discuss the impact of the disease on the patient and I have invited three patients to participate in our discussion." He turned towards the right side of the stage and said, "Will you bring on our guests please."

Three patients in pajamas and gown maneuvered their wheelchairs on stage.

"Our guests know their diagnosis and they know that their chances of surviving their disease are extremely small," Dameshek continued. "This means that their priorities are now different from ours and I want you to remember that at all times when you are caring for your patients. Our common day-to-day concerns are no longer theirs. Take for instance the daily news; that probably is no longer interesting to them?"

"You're wrong, doctor," a pale emaciated young man in the middle wheelchair interrupted the great professor. "I read the New York Times every day and I look at the news on TV."

"Me too," the woman next to him said firmly. "I also want to hear what's going on."

The third patient, a middle-aged man who looked distinguished despite the pajamas and gown, turned to the audience. "I am a banker and I must have my Wall Street Journal. I think that we all three are more interested in the news than we were before we became ill. We do not wish to be written off by our family and friends before we die. Reading and listening to the news keeps us informed. That may perhaps surprise some of you, but you must remember that we are still here. We are still alive."

A dumbfounded Dameshek broke the silence that followed. "This may be a good time for questions from the audience." The lecture became a lively give and take between audience and patients, something none of us would forget. Life indeed continues remarkably well when family and friends continue to include the patient in everything, and I mean everything. We should never exclude the patient from our discussions and from decision-making. They are part of us and we best not forget that.

Dameshek would have really been surprised by what had happened to me a few years earlier.

"It's disgusting," the middle-aged nurse burst out as she walked into the nursing station.

"What's the matter," her supervisor asked.

"A guy is raping that poor girl in 467. I'm going to call the police."

The supervisor looked at me with a face like 'Do something.'

"You mean they are having sex?" I asked the agitated nurse.

"That's not sex, that's rape. That girl is helpless."

"That girl is seventeen and that guy as you call him is her boy friend."

"How do you know?"

"I know because I saw them and I closed her door to give them privacy."

"Well doctor, then you're even more disgusting, filthy." She spit the words at me.

"Alright Mrs. Browning, now you listen to me. That girl is my patient. She has acute leukemia and has very few days left to live. What you in your narrow mind call rape, is to me the most beautiful expression of life I have ever witnessed. She knows that she is going to die soon and so does her boy friend. If you cannot understand that their moment of intimacy is beautiful, then I pity you. Now pick up that damn phone and call your police if you want, but I never again want you come even close to my patients."

"That'll be fine with me, *doctor*." She stomped to the elevator.

"The bitch," said the supervisor. "Thank you, doctor. That was telling her."

Much has been written about sexual problems of patients with cancer. The articles describe the impact of self-esteem on sexual function and psychosocial issues such as guilt feeling. I have yet to read an article about the desire for sex in our patients with late stage cancer. Oncologists should not hesitate to discuss it with their patients, and, when the love between two partners reaches that moment of expression, facilitate it. If necessary, find an empty private room, close the door and let them express their love.

13

NIENKE AND OUR FAMILY

Nienke stayed home, had children, and cared for them while I tried to build a career, which often involved travel. Evelien was born in Valhalla Hospital in Westchester County, New York, when we lived in the two rooms in Elmsford. She was the quietest baby one could imagine, and she had the worst possible pigeon-toes. Her little feet were so turned inside that her big toes said hello to each other. The orthopedist advised us to wait until she was six months old before fitting her with a steel bar with shoes at the ends. This contraption fixed her little feet with the toes turned all the way outward. She wore it day and night for the next nine months. Eve took it like a real trooper; she never cried. She managed to hoist herself up on the side of her crib and stood for hours, and instead of crawling she pulled herself forward on her stomach. However, the bar forced Nienke to carry her wherever they went, which was not easy when she was pregnant again.

"Frank had his polio shot today," Nienke said one day when I got home. "And you know he said 'thank you' after the doctor gave him the injection. You should have seen the face of that doctor."

We were fortunate to have our apartment on Warburton Avenue in Yonkers, opposite the school and Trevor Park along the Hudson River. When the sun came up in the morning it highlighted the Palisades on the other side of the river and in the evening its last rays played through the treetops. The apartment had a kitchen, a living room, three small bedrooms and a bathroom. We were rich. We were so rich that after we spent nearly ten dollars to buy groceries Nienke had seven cents left. That was it, seven cents to last for three weeks while I waited for my first paycheck from Mount Sinai.

When Nienke came home from shopping, she first carried Eve up the sixteen high stone steps alongside the garage. Behind her Frank slowly and manfully climbed one step at the time. Next came twelve steps to the house, and then fifteen steps to the second floor, forty-three steps in all. After she put Eve in the crib, Nien walked down to the street level, picked up the groceries, and walked back up. She traveled by bus, because I needed our car.

Snow fell in March 1960 when she went to the hospital for the delivery. "Make sure that they call me in time, I want to be there," I said.

A nurse called two hours later to say that there had been no progress and that Nienke was sound asleep. I took Frank and Evelien for a sled ride down the steep slope of the park. It was beautiful outside and we were the first ones to go down.

"Daddy will go first and make a trail. You wait here."

Down I went on my stomach. The sled gathered speed, hit a large hidden rock, and I somersaulted through the air. Remembering my early Jiu Jitsu training, I tried to break the fall, only to fracture my left arm in the process. I picked up the sled and trudged back up the slope.

"Now me, now me," yelled Frank.

"Me," echoed Eve.

"Daddy hurt his arm," I said through clenched teeth. "We'll go another day."

Deeply disappointed, they trudged behind me. A neighbor took care of the children while I went to the hospital in Yonkers where the best orthopedist in town put the arm in a cast and told me to come back in six weeks. At one o'clock a nurse called. "Doctor, we tried to call you earlier. Your wife had a baby girl."

Poor Nienke had gone through it all alone. Two days later I saw the newly appointed chairman of Orthopedics at Mount Sinai. He looked at a new X-ray, removed the cast, and gave me a sling to wear. "Go home and exercise that elbow under water and don't come back," he advised. Two weeks later the arm was as good as new.

Nienke had a one-armed chauffeur when she came home with Marion, the latest addition to our growing family. Somehow she managed to take care of a house and three young children, and after I returned from a trip to Japan she became pregnant once more. While her parents lived on Java in Indonesia, their only son was killed in a car accident when he was ten years old, and deep in her heart Nienke was afraid; she wanted another boy.

After she became pregnant again, Nienke came to me with a proposition. "I'd like to go to Holland for the delivery," she said, "But then you're alone again."

Our apartment was not air-conditioned and I hated to see her go through a hot summer with a baby expected in July. "Look, I can manage. It's you I'm worried about. You already have your hands full with the other kids. I'm sure your mother would love to have you and that your Dad will spoil them rotten. Go."

So Nienke and the children left for Holland, where our fourth child was born on July 26. After six months in Holland, she flew back to the States with four children aged six, three, one year and a newborn, Nick Rudolph, and, our apartment was now too small. We looked for another place and found a house at 32

Poplar Street in Portchester. It was just the kind of house and location Nienke needed. Across the street, a few sheep and a Brahman bull grazed on a meadow that had once been part of a large estate. The children loved those animals, especially when the sheep came closer to nibble on grass hesitantly offered through the fence by a child's hand. One block up was Lyons Park, which had once been part of the farm, as most of the neighborhood had been. The park was a safe haven for mothers with small children. There they could roam at will, slide the slides and swing the swings.

Beyond the park was King Street School, where Mr. deBono ruled his flock. It was a public school that was as good as any private school. Former students best remember deBono for his ten-second rule at the water fountain. While one student drank, the next in line counted off the seconds. A quick last sip at ten and turn away with water dripping down the chin, so that the floor around the fountain was always wet. The school band was the best in the city. Frank played the trombone, Evelien the flute, Marion the saxophone, and Nick couldn't carry a tune. The band was so good that it was invited to play in the Rose Bowl Parade. Never before had so many cars needed unnecessary washings, were so many chocolates and cookies eaten and so many lawns mowed, because most parents insisted that their children pay part of the costs.

A week before the band departed for California, the members paraded through town in spanking new uniforms. The whole town was glued to television sets on that second day in January and cheered, "There they are!" when our band came on the screen. Seven trombones led the way with the tallest boy, Frank, in the middle, his eyes fixed in the yellow line in the center of the street. They marched proudly behind a large group of horses, and when we all saw Frank take an awkward step to avoid a fresh dropping, we all laughed.

For their fiftieth wedding anniversary Nienke's parents were scheduled to visit us in Port Chester and that presented a problem. They were used to the short distances in Holland and did not have the slightest idea how big our adopted country was. Nienke always maintained that her eyes were not good enough to drive a car and, being the stubborn Friesian that she was, she would not take lessons from me. I resorted to subterfuge. One day she answered the doorbell to a stranger.

"Good morning, Mrs. Hoogstraten; I am your instructor."

"My instructor? What are you talking about?"

"I am here to give you your first driving lesson."

There was no escape, and she became a good driver. Her parents came over by boat, and the children immediately called them Oma and Grova to distinguish them from my parents, who were Grandpa and Grandma. With Nienke driving a new Ford station wagon, they explored southern New England, the beaches, the supermarkets, and the Untermeyer Estate. Grova made a real piece of art of the Halloween pumpkin to the delight of the children, who insisted that they had the best pumpkin in the neighborhood. Oma made the costumes, but not for poor Nick, who as the last of the children inherited the Mickey Mouse outfit that Nienke had originally made for Frank.

It was hard to tell who spoiled whom the most, the grandparents who had not seen the little ones in years or the children who doted on Oma and Grova. Now they too had grandparents, just like other children. In the morning they brought them tea with biscuits in bed, they sat on laps, held hands while walking through cornfields, did all those things only little children and old people do together, and their happiness made their faces even more beautiful. They raked the leaves in the fall and shoveled snow in the winter. In the supermarket they used two carts so that Marion and Nick could both get a ride. The wedding anniversary was a great success, Christmas came and went, and Nienke and I danced with the old folks on New Years Eve. Too soon, the six months went by and Oma and Grova had a new adventure; they flew back to Holland.

My parents came over in 1966, and it was in Port Chester, New York, of all places that dad completed his last work. Before leaving Holland, he asked if there was anything we wanted done to our house. He didn't want to be bored. An enclosed porch to the side of our brick house was made of wood and connected by two archways to the living room. We thought it would look nice if its walls were also made of brick. When Dad boarded the plane the stewardess was puzzled by the strange package he carried.

"What is that?" she asked.

It was his old mortarboard.

Dad had a good look at the house before he entered. "Harvard brick. Your house is built with Harvard brick."

I was dumbfounded. He had never been in the States and the first thing he says is that these were Harvard bricks. How on earth did he know?

"You know it or you don't," was all Dad said.

The next day I called every building supply company in the telephone book and only two had heard of Harvard bricks, but they did not have them. One dealer said that they hadn't been made in a long time. Father Gijs started to nose around on his own, and on the third day he announced that the bricks and other building material would be delivered the next day. The store manager accompanied the delivery truck. He told me the following tale.

> It was the darndest thing I've ever experienced in my life. This old man came in the store, he didn't speak English and just started talking in a language I had never heard before. The only word I understood was "Harvard" and he pointed to a brick. I motioned that we didn't have those bricks and then, on his own, he walked all over the back yard. After a while he came back in the office, took me by the arm, and walked me to the far corner of the yard. Hidden under sand and partially overgrown with grass was a heap of bricks, which he indicated were Harvard bricks. I never knew that they were there, but he sure wanted them. He then proceeded to take me through the rest of the place and indicated what else he needed, like sand, bags of cement, four-by-fours, boards, nails; you name it, and you know something? We got along fine. In the end I made out the bill and he scribbled his name on it. He pointed out that I had not priced the brick, but I told him that it was a present from me to him. Actually I was glad to get rid of them. They are something else, those people from the old country. Your dad is quite a man.

Dad donned the gray overalls he brought along from Holland and went to work. He put supports under the ceiling and roof of the twenty by ten-foot porch and removed the walls, but saved the window frames because they were going back in later. Gijs was in his element. He dug holes for the foundation, evened out the ground, added a layer of gravel, and fashioned a network of reinforced steel over it. He put cement on top of the network, and, while that was drying, he began putting up the walls. A city building inspector came by to see what was going on, and he and Dad struck up quite a conversation, short on words, but long on gestures. In the end they slapped each other on the shoulder.

"The manager of the store told me about your old man, and I had to come and see for myself," he said. "He sure knows what he is doing."

"What were you two talking about so long?" I asked.

"About the old country. My Dad came over from Germany and he too was a bricklayer. If you don't mind, I asked your Dad over for a beer come next Saturday. He and my old man will have a ball."

That is how Dad made friends in a strange country, not speaking the language, by just being himself. While Dad worked, Mom looked on and handed him a hammer or whatever. In the evening they played klaverjassen, a popular card game in Holland and Belgium. Dad—his fingers stiff and gnarled—bent the cards and Mom straightened them. Near the end of their visit they knew the back of every card in the deck, but it did not seem to matter. Mom did some knitting and helped out with the dishes. Dad took out his pocketknife and fashioned a doll or toy for the children from leftover wood. Without knowing the rules of the game, they liked football and basketball on TV, but they missed soccer. Baseball and golf were too slow. "Person can fall asleep watching that," Mother said.

We brought them to the airport. "That's enough travel for us. From now on you have to come to Holland if you want to see us," Dad said.

Our children still remember the wooden toys.

The deaths of our parents were difficult for us. Nienke left in time to spend two weeks of precious time at her father's bedside, but she was too late when her mother died. Her sister called every day with a progress report and Nienke was ready to leave at a moment's notice, but the end came too suddenly. I was not prepared when my dad died. My brother Jaap kept me informed and I frequently called the nursing station. The patient rooms didn't have phones. "He had a good day, doctor," the nurse said.

"Dad died this afternoon," Jaap called at about eight that same evening.

"Dad is dead," I said to Nienke.

I went to our bedroom, sat on the side of the bed and cried. I couldn't stop, face in the pillow to drown the sound. I kept seeing his hands with the thick calluses, the nails that did not need clipping—the bricks and the mortar kept them short. The years of holding the two by two-foot board loaded with mortar above his head with one hand and the heavy trowel in the other, which made it impossible for him to straighten his fingers, and he couldn't make a fist. Pieces of callus peeled from the palms of his hands to expose pink rawness. Moisture crept through the cracks in the callus and fungus followed. "Cement rot," he called it. Dirty bandages covered part of the pink. Black electric insulation strips hid the tips of some fingers. They were the hands of a master bricklayer and plasterer, my dad's hands.

There was no way I was going to miss Mother's last days. Again it was Jaap who kept me informed. I was supposed to chair an important meeting that week and called the doctor at his home in Hilversum. It was nine o'clock in the evening there, and his wife answered.

"I am Dr. Hoogstraten, calling from America. Can I talk to your husband please?"

"My husband is not at home."

"He is my mother's physician and I'll appreciate it very much if he could call me back tonight. Can you please leave the message?"

"No, I will not. It is my husband's day off and I will not disturb him." She was adamant.

"But I'm calling from America and need to know when I should come over."

"You can call him in his office tomorrow," and she hung up.

God did that made me angry. Had the practice of medicine in Holland deteriorated so far that doctors worked by the hour? Did they no longer have the decency to call a faraway daughter or son, not even a colleague? When I called his office the next morning, the nurse said that he would not be in that day. I called Jaap instead. "I think you should come," he said.

I went and the three of us had two valuable days together. The funeral was a reunion, with uncles, aunts, cousins, and with nieces and nephews I did not know I had. Today Nienke's sister and Jaap are the last threads binding us to Holland.

14

THE ACADEMIC SUICIDE

In many ways, the academic world is not much different from the business world. Like some business executives, some ambitious scientists forget all forms of decency and will do anything to get ahead in their profession, even if that means climbing over the backs of their colleagues. They're too impatient to wait for top positions to open up; they want them now, no matter at whose expense. Victor Herbert was such a person.

Victor had worked with Wasserman before I came to Sinai. On Lou's recommendation, he left for Boston to work under Professor William Castle at Harvard, where he was in competition with Dr. James Jandl, a lanky New Englander whose main research interest was in iron metabolism. It was no big secret that after Castle retired, these two would vie for the chair of medicine.

In 1962 Wasserman looked for a second in command. Richard Rosenfield would have been an excellent choice, but Dick, a world power in blood banking, had no interest in the job. I was still one of the lesser lights in the department at the time.

Lou brought Victor back. He gave him a large laboratory and began to nurture him as his possible successor. Vic's major interest was in folic acid metabolism. In October 1961, he put himself on a folic acid free diet; no fresh fruit, no vegetables, and everything cooked until there was no trace of folic acid left. It was a miserable diet. He began to lose weight, had diarrhea and headaches, and after four months he became increasingly fatigued. He had numerous blood counts done, examined his blood weekly for the level of folic acid, and his friend, Dr. Ralph Zalusky, performed several bone marrow aspirations on him. When he developed signs of megaloblastic anemia and had lost twenty-six pounds, he had proven his point. It was indeed a heroic effort, and he received a well-deserved standing ovation from his peers when he presented the results at the 1962 Federation Meetings in Atlantic City. Thanks to him, folic acid is now a required additive to all American food grains.

Victor had a habit I found annoying. During the weekly Thursday morning conferences he like to comment on presentations and back it up by adding, "You will find it in the July issue of the New England Journal, page 228, second paragraph," or a similar reference. It impressed everybody, but the speakers and listeners did not always appreciate it. After he corrected a distinguished guest speaker and quoted a journal and page, I left the room, found the journal, and confronted him. "Here is the journal and what you just quoted isn't in it."

"It must be in another issue," he tried to shrug it off. "I'll show you later."

However, he didn't and he made fewer references after that. During the Christmas party later that year Victor jokingly promoted me to Shabbos Goy. Each week the Jewish Sabbath starts at sundown on Fridays and lasts until sundown on Saturday. During these twenty-four hours the orthodox Jews are not allowed to perform any work, not even turn on a lamp. A Shabbos goy is a non-Jew paid to do the work for them during that time. There were no ill feelings between Victor and me.

As part of his research he took portions of the small bowel of rats, turned them inside out and exposed these "inverted sacs" to radioactive folic acid. He could now demonstrate how fast, how much, and in which portion of the bowel folic acid was absorbed. It was an ingenious invention and he was rightfully proud of it. He even obtained a patent for it. However, one day he came to me with an article in a Dutch magazine, *Het Nederlandse Tijdschrift van Geneeskunde*, and asked me to translate it. Professor Henk Nieweg of the University of Groningen described in detail a new method to study absorption by the intestine. It was all about the "inverted sac" and was a blow to Victor, who had yet to publish his findings.

"I presented it at a meeting before this article came out," he said.

"Where did you present it, Victor?" I asked, as if I did not know.

"At the Academy of Medicine."

"That was not an officially recognized meeting, Vic."

He sold his patent to Sinai for one dollar. When in 1982, I was invited to give a lecture at the University of Groningen, I told Henk about the episode over a drink. He just smiled. It often goes that way in science. You work on something for a long time, finally succeed, and then find out that someone else has published it before you. Victor received well-deserved accolades for his work, though.

The 1982 annual meeting of the American Society of Hematology took place in Toronto. The chairman of the plenary session, the aforementioned Professor William Castle, introduced the session's guest speaker, Victor, who gave a brilliant talk on the interrelationship between folic acid and vitamin B_{12}. After he finished, Castle announced that he had granted a request from Dr. Luhby to give a five-minute rebuttal. Luhby worked in a hospital six blocks north of Sinai and he too studied folic acid, but his was crude research. He went well over his allotted five minutes and the huge audience began to get restless.

"I better stop here, because I see that Professor Castle is getting itchy," he finally said.

"Yes Dr. Luhby, I was getting itchy, but I didn't scratch," Bill replied ever so dryly to a standing ovation.

Under the leadership of the Chairman of the Board, Gus Levy, Mount Sinai became a medical school and the first Dean was a man with no experience in academia, Dr. George James, the former New York City Commissioner of Health. They gave him a huge office on the top floor of one of the many buildings overlooking Central Park and a desk the likes of which nobody had ever seen. It was an enormous semi-circular monstrosity covered with a two-inch thick marble slab. About eight chairs were arranged on the outside of the semi-circle and the Dean's chair was on the inside. He also had a conference room with a large table, also covered with marble. You didn't dare lean on the table because it was so darn cold. Everything was cold in that place.

The Board also selected Dr. Sol Berson as the new chairman and professor of Medicine. Berson came from the Veterans Administration Hospital in the Bronx, where, together with his associate Dr. Rosalyn S. Yalow, he did important research. Had he lived long enough, Yalow would have shared her Nobel Prize for Medicine with him. At his investiture as the new chairman, James proudly listed Berson's many virtues. "Not only is Dr. Berson a brilliant researcher and a superb teacher, but he is also a fine violinist. I know; I heard him play. And on top of that he is a master chess player."

I sat in the back next to the Bader twins, both avid chess players.

"We'll have to see about that, Barth," Richard whispered.

Berson had no experience in dealing with the powerful private practice physicians who ruled Mount Sinai. He was a newcomer to the intense politics that always boil in large hospitals, especially in those connected with medical schools. As a result, he banged his head a couple of times when he moved full steam ahead without consulting with a few insiders first. If he had done so, he would have avoided the Victor Herbert disaster that became a blemish on Mount Sinai and on himself.

The background to the story began two years earlier during a meeting on the boardwalk of Atlantic City. Wasserman invited me to a lunch with Bill and while those two giants talked, I kept quiet. We left the restaurant and walked slowly back to the convention hall in the bright sunshine of the early summer. Dameshek suddenly said, "You know what the trouble is with your department Lou? You have no serious research."

That stung. Louis R. Wasserman was proud of his department. He wanted it to be the best in the world and it was one of the best. He did not reply, but back in Mount Sinai he found more laboratory space and then successfully wooed Dr. Charlotte Friend to move her leukemia virus research program from Sloan-Kettering to Mount Sinai, where he built a modern and very expensive laboratory to her specifications.

After Berson arrived, Victor quickly gained his confidence and the two began to scheme. Berson wanted hematology to become a division in his department and Victor could not wait for his boss to reach the mandatory retirement age. I got an inkling that something was brewing when I received a call from Dr. Stan Steckler, the director of medicine at Elmhurst Hospital.

"Barth, I would I like you to talk to you. Can you come to my office?"

"Why don't you come down to my office, Stan?"

From the tone of his voice I had a feeling that it was better to talk on my territory. Stan came down.

"I would like you to become part of the Department of Medicine," he said. "With your expertise in clinical research and standing in hematology, you'll be a tribute to the medicine department here."

His offer came out of the blue.

"Let me think it over Stan, and I'll let you know."

I would not have minded joining him, but such a big change needed Wasserman's approval, and he was out of the country. At the request of the NIH he had just begun a speaking tour to several countries overseas.

That same afternoon my phone rang again. It was Victor.

"Barth, did Stan Steckler talk to you?"

"Yes he did."

"Well, what do you think?"

"I think I better talk it over with Dr. Wasserman."

"Oh you don't have to worry about Lou. Sol Berson will take good care of you. We'll protect you."

"Protect me from what, Victor? I have never talked with Berson, but it looks to me that he is behind all this and he should be doing his own calling and not use you."

"He will. Stay close to the phone. He'll call you right back."

Berson did no such thing.

What was going on? What was that "protection" business? Why on Earth would I need protection from Wasserman, my mentor, the man who brought me along and had helped me with my career? I trusted Lou Wasserman implicitly. I smelled a rat. Something rotten was going on with Wasserman out of the country and I called Dick Rosenfield.

"Dick, something funny is going on and I don't like it."

I explained what had happened and he agreed with me.

"Let me do some investigating and I'll be in touch."

Later that day we agreed that Wasserman had to come back immediately and we would both try to get in touch with him. I reached him in Luxembourg.

"Lou, don't ask any questions," I said. "Just get back here as fast as you can, otherwise you won't have a department when you come back."

It was the first time I ever called him by his first name. While Wasserman and his wife Julia took the next plane back to New York, Dick and I did our homework. It turned out that Victor had written a letter to the dean in which he attacked his boss and he sent a copy of the letter to Berson and to Associate Dean Hans Popper, but not to Martin Steinberg, the longtime director of Mount Sinai Hospital and good friend of Louis Wasserman. With his boss safely out of the country, Victor figured that this was the time to act. He obviously had the backing of Berson, but had not counted on our loyalty.

I did not know that the Wassermans were back in the country until Dick called me at home. It was Saturday evening. "James has called a meeting for tomorrow morning in his office. Can you be there?"

"Sure, but what about Lou?"

"He's back."

I called him at home.

"Everything is OK. I'll take care of the situation," he said.

I was furious and exploded; "You bastard, how the hell do you think you can take care of it alone? We are sticking our necks out and you will do it alone? Well go ahead and see where it gets you."

I hung up. Never before had I talked to him like that. Immediately the phone rang a second time. "Can you please come over now?"

He looked tired when he opened the door to his apartment. I was close to tears when he led me into the small side room he used as an office.

"Damn it, you're like a second father to me. You must let us help you," I said in a choked voice.

"I will and I'm very grateful to you. Only good friends can hurt each other the way I have hurt you." His voice wasn't so solid either.

Dick, who had been in another room, walked in and we made plans together. Dean James had called a meeting for ten o'clock Sunday morning, and we made sure that as many staff members as possible would attend on such short notice. Dick and I would be the frontmen. After that meeting, James was scheduled to meet with Steinberg, Popper, and Berson. Dick had alerted Steinberg and had obtained a copy of the soon-to-be infamous letter from Popper. Victor not only wanted Wasserman's job as director of hematology, he also wanted to get his hands on the large fund that Wasserman was supposed to have stashed away somewhere; however, when he went through Wasserman's papers, he couldn't find it. In the letter he accused Wasserman of both embezzlement and a reign of tyranny within the division. "The Russians in the concentration camps under Stalin fared better than the fellows and staff do under Wasserman." The long letter ended with the recommendation that Dr. Wasserman be removed as head of the division and that, while the charges against Wasserman were being investigated, he, Victor Herbert, was willing to act as the interim head.

A good dean would demand that all copies of the letter be turned over to him or her. He would have told Herbert to pipe down and keep his mouth shut while he waited until Wasserman returned from his trip. But not James. He called the meetings without first investigating what was going on. Herbert was already in the conference room when we entered. James welcomed us with a nod and took a chair at the head of the table. He invited Victor to sit next to him and the eight of us tried not to touch the marble. James opened the session.

"I have asked you to come here on short notice because Dr. Herbert has expressed serious concerns about the Division of Hematology and I need to know how widespread that concern is."

That did not exactly sound like he was completely neutral. It was as if he already accepted that there were reasons for concern.

"I have asked Dr. Herbert to make an opening statement and then we will go around the table for your comments."

Victor put on a serious, almost somber face and began by saying that he had written a letter to the Dean after he found out that a large sum of money was missing from division funds. He followed this with a long harangue about the working conditions within the division under Wasserman's leadership and made the comparison with Stalin and the concentration camps. He even had the audacity to repeat his recommendation that Wasserman be temporarily removed as the head of the division. I noticed that he already used the word *division* instead of *department*.

Herbert was right in one aspect; it was not always easy to work for LRW and I had also had a few run-ins with him. During Grand Rounds one time I corrected him when I knew that he had badly misquoted something. "In my office," he growled at me at the end of Rounds. In the office, he lashed out at me and—as always when he was angry—he went on and on for ten or twenty minutes. "I have enough people sticking knives in my back," he snarled.

"In the front," I finally interrupted.

"What the hell are you saying?" He leaned forward.

"I'm saying that you're wrong. I stuck the knife in front."

That made him think for a moment, and then the grin appeared and the outburst was over.

Herbert continued. "As second in command, I am the logical person to take over as the interim director until Dr. Berson has had a chance to appoint a new head," he added with a little smile.

Herbert was pretty sure that Berson would be in the position to appoint a new head of hematology. Neither he nor James knew that Dick and I had already read a copy of the letter. As Victor made his speech, the others around the table became wide-eyed with amazement. Someone whispered "Wow!" Another blew his cheeks out and slowly let the air slip away. A third leaned back and surreptitiously looked around to see how the others reacted. One man put the palms of his hands before his face with the index fingers against his nose and stared at a spot on the ceiling. I kept my eyes on Herbert.

"Aren't you running a little ahead of yourself?" Rosenfield said dryly.

James went around the table. He only addressed Dick by name and pointed to the others as "You." He had not bothered to ask us to identify ourselves. Most people had little or nothing to say. Only one person agreed that the atmosphere within the division was not always pleasant.

It was Dick's turn. "How do you know that funds are missing? You must have rifled through Wasserman's files while he was somewhere in Europe."

"Why did you wait until Dr. Wasserman was out of the country to write that letter?" Janet Cuttner wanted to know.

Victor responded by saying that he had a large bill to pay and that was when he found out about the missing money. He evidently did not know, as Dick and I did, that Wasserman had laid out six hundred thousand dollars to build Charlotte's new laboratory. Victor smiled rather faintly and began to sweat, the smelly kind of sweat.

"Where is your sense of loyalty?" I asked when it was my turn. "And what is that nonsense about comparing hematology to a Russian concentration camp?"

"Barth, you yourself told me at the last Christmas party that it was hell to work under Wasserman." He was now on the defensive.

"Victor, you're both a liar and a coward."

"Well, I may be wrong about it. Maybe I was too drunk at the time."

He laughed sickly, but he had made a big mistake by retreating instead of continuing the attack. Soon thereafter James thanked us for coming and the meeting broke up. Popper, Steinberg and Wasserman were waiting outside when we left the room. However, Berson, the man who had been behind the power grab from the beginning, was strangely absent. I don't know what went on during that second meeting, but the outcome was that Wasserman became an even stronger figure at Mount Sinai Hospital. Herbert was permanently exiled to the VA hospital. He never set foot in hematology again as long as Wasserman was the director.

Something as serious as this was does not remain a secret very long. Victor was never invited to become the chairman of a department in another medical school; he never became the head of a reputable division. That was a shame, because he was an outstanding hematologist, a top nutrition scientist and the recipient of several awards. He was a brilliant man, but he could not wait his turn. He committed academic suicide. What a waste.

To set the record straight, James ordered Berson to meet with each member of the hematology staff individually. He called me last.

"Doctor Hoogstraten, I'd like see you early tomorrow morning. Say at five o'clock?"

If he had said three o'clock I would have been there. Later that day he changed the time of our meeting to nine o'clock. Meanwhile I called Elliott Osserman, who I knew to be a friend of Berson.

"Elliott, what kind of man is Sol Berson?" I asked.

"He is a straight shooter, Barth."

The next morning Berson let me cool my heels for nearly an hour before his secretary finally said that I could go in. We did not shake hands.

"Doctor Berson, Elliott Osserman tells me that you are a straight shooter," I opened before he had a chance.

"Yes I am."

"Then why were you in such a hurry that your arrow came off crooked?"

It was a short conversation, but it was not the last time that Sol Berson and I went head to head. A myth was about to be exposed thanks to the Bader twins.

Every year during the Federation meetings in Atlantic City, Wasserman took the entire hematology staff to dinner, and I had quite a number of drinks that evening. A message waited for me when I came back in my hotel room. "Please come to our room for a game of chess," signed, Mortimer. He opened the door when I arrived and those two rascals had a surprise waiting for me in the persons of Drs. Berson and Yalow.

"Barth, why don't you play a game with Sol?"

The board was already set up and waiting. The twins took lessons from Pal Benko, an international grandmaster, and they were good players. I was a member of the Manhattan Chess Club and played against masters, including Bobby Fischer, who twice wiped the floor with me. Berson opened pawn E4 and he played fast. He tried a cheap trap that didn't work and lost in less than five minutes. In the second game he was more careful and I had to concentrate through the slight haze of alcohol. He lost again in about fifteen minutes.

"OK, now I know at what level you play and we'll have a serious game," he said, intent to teach me a lesson. However, he did not have the patience to think out problem situations. Just like in his abortive attempt to take over the hematology department, he was in too much of a hurry and lost. Berson was neither a master chess player, nor a master plotter.

"We'll have to play again some time," he said.

We never did. The twins loved to talk and the truth about the master chess player spread fast across the boardwalk the next day. Wasserman loved it. I was sure Berson wouldn't forget it.

Not long thereafter Berson learned another lesson about politics in Mount Sinai.

"Barth, you're a member of the Cancer Committee, aren't you?" Wasserman asked over the phone.

"I am? I didn't even know that there was such a committee."

"Well there is now, and you are on it. This afternoon at two there is a meeting in Steinberg's office. Be there."

He did not explain what the sudden meeting was about, but knowing him it had to be important. The chairmen of all the clinical departments were present at the meeting. Dr. Ezra Greenspan and I were the only nonchairmen. John Boland, the chairman of the Radiation Therapy Department, opened the meeting.

"I have called this meeting of the Cancer Committee to hear an important proposal from Dr. Berson. Sol, why don't tell the committee what you have in mind."

Berson stood and began: "As you all know, important progress is being made in the treatment of cancer and I think that Mount Sinai should be at the forefront of these new developments. I propose that we form an interdepartmental division for cancer therapy and I know of no better man to head such division than Ezra Greenspan." He sat down.

He had never had anything to do with cancer, but in two sentences he not only proposed a plan that would have far-reaching implications for every department in the hospital but also told us who should lead the program. Now it was clear why the meeting was held in Steinberg's office and not upstairs in the Dean's quarters. This was friendly territory. An icy silence fell over the room. John Boland, an Englishman, studied the desk in front of him. The ceiling lamps also received a lot of attention. Somebody had to say something, but nobody did. Finally Berson himself broke the silence.

"Dr. Greenspan, why don't you explain what you and I have been talking about."

That was the giveaway: "You and I." Once again Berson hadn't done his homework. He had not discussed the proposal with his colleagues and had not lined up any support behind his proposal. Poor Ezra had to follow his masters' begging. At the start of his career, he had done some fine work at the National Cancer Institute and he was probably the first man to treat cancer with a combination of drugs. He was genuinely interested in cancer, had a thriving private practice in that field and with his own money operated a small research laboratory.

"I think that we ought to combine our efforts and the best way to do that is by forming a cancer division." He said and sat down. Unlike Berson, Ezra was familiar with the power politics of Mount Sinai.

"Can we hear from the committee members about the proposal?" Boland came alive.

Saul Gusberg, chairman of OB-GYN, a polite, gentle man, who despite his friendly appearance could cut a person down to size like no other, was the first to respond. "I think it's an excellent idea, Sol. Of course, you realize that we already have an ongoing program in GYN. Our service is unique in that it only involves a relatively small part of the body and only women. I'm sure you understand that we cannot get involved with your proposal at the present time."

It was such a nice way of brushing him off. Next came the Chairman of surgery, a South African. He too complimented Berson on his idea and he too said that he could not participate. John Boland drove the nail in further.

"Radiation therapy is a highly specialized and fully developed specialty. We already hold joint clinics with Hematology. Perhaps Dr. Greenspan would like to join us."

Wasserman, who had kept quiet through it all, now said, "Barth, why don't you explain the situation in Hematology."

So that's why you wanted me to come to this meeting, I thought. Although he was not afraid of anybody, Lou thought it better not to tangle with Berson a second time.

"Well, as you know, in Hematology we are only concerned with the leukemias, multiple myeloma and the lymphomas. We are fully committed to the studies of the Acute Leukemia Group B and cannot be distracted from that program. Perhaps Ezra can start something in the Department of Medicine by concentrating on the solid tumors and when he is successful, we can talk about a combined program some years from now." It was the best I could do, diplomatically speaking.

Boland had the last word. "There appears to be a consensus that each department will continue to develop its own program. Sol, thank you for bringing up an interesting proposal. The meeting is adjourned."

It was all very neat and very clean. Not a drop of blood spilled—a fast kill, stiletto style. Never before had I witnessed how efficiently the department chairmen could cut a major medical school figure down to size. They left Berson standing in his underwear and there wasn't a thing he could do about it. Was this otherwise brilliant man, though not in chess and perhaps not on the violin, really so dumb as to think that he could pull off this stunt or did he decide beforehand. that Gusberg, Boland and the chairman of surgery would reject the whole idea and that it was only a ploy to get Hematology under his control? Had he hoped that those three would volunteer a suggestion that Hematology, meaning Wasserman, join forces with him, in which case Wasserman would have been in an awkward position? Even if that was the case, he should have known that he was the new kid on the block, so to speak, and that the others would never let Wasserman down. True, Lou could be nasty at times and had battled with every one of them. However, Berson had yet to learn that Louis R. Wasserman was a man of his word, a man who over the years had done a lot for Mount Sinai and had been a superb host to all of them.

"When did you learn that you are the chairman of the Cancer Committee?" I asked John Boland on the way out.

"This morning, as a matter of fact," the Englishman replied with typically dry British understatement.

When Dr. Victor Daniel Herbert died on November 19, 2002, at age seventy-five, there was a well-deserved obituary in *The New York Times* comprising three columns and photograph.

Sol Berson never entered the inner circle of power at Mount Sinai. A few years later he dropped dead from a heart attack while jogging on the boardwalk in Atlantic City. Dean James was not long for this world either. A saying started making the rounds at Mount Sinai: "It isn't nice to fool with Lou Wasserman." Lou helped recruit the director of the Clinical Center of the National Institutes of Health, Thomas C. Chalmers, as the new dean. When Wasserman himself retired, he recommended an excellent hematologist as the new director for the Division of Hematology and he was instrumental in persuading James Holland to come to Sinai as the first chairman of the newly formed Department of Neoplastic Diseases, the first such department in the country.

Wasserman was recognized worldwide for his studies of red cell metabolism; he was president of the American Society of Hematology, vice president of the International Society of Hematology and chairman of the Board of Scientific Counselors of the Division of Cancer Treatment of the NCI. Louis Robert Wasserman died on June 21, 1999, at age eighty-eight. A small man with a strong personality and an explosive temper, he was a dominating figure wherever he went. He was a most gracious host and a generous man, whose gruffness hid his shyness. That man was my mentor for twelve years and he made it possible for me to succeed. I loved that man who was so hard to love.

Nienke and I best remember him for his annual faculty outings on his farm in Connecticut. He would show up on a tractor with a long cart behind it. The kids climbed aboard and off they went. They laughed and squealed and yelled, "Look Mommy, Dad, hey Dad!" and Lou had a big happy smile on his face. There was no photograph with his obituary in *The New York Times*.

15

THE UNIVERSITY OF KANSAS MEDICAL CENTER

Sometime in November 1969, Nienke and I went to a concert in New York City.

"This is filthy," she remarked as we drove through Manhattan.

"What do you mean, filthy?"

"The streets are filthy. There is garbage everywhere. How can you stand it?"

She was right, the streets *were* filthy, and I was so used to it that I no longer noticed. I could not keep my mind on the music during the concert. Why did I waste so much time on the New York Thruway each day? Did I really enjoy my work? Was I in a rut? Maybe it was time to move on?

"I am going to leave you," I told a surprised Wasserman the next morning.

"That's rather sudden, isn't it?"

"Yes. I made up my mind last night."

"Where are you going?"

"I don't know."

"You mean to tell me that you are leaving without having a job lined up?"

"Well, I think it's only fair that you hear it from me first."

"I appreciate that and wish you luck," he said abruptly. He didn't ask why I was leaving him. He probably realized it was time for me to go out on my own.

One does not advertise for a job in the academe; nor does it advertise. I had been with Wasserman so long that it was assumed that I was going to stay with him permanently, that I was an untouchable. It was only through the grapevine that people learned that I was available. Feelers soon came from several places, but Nienke and I had our own agenda. Chicago was out because it was just another large city. Los Angeles experienced one of its thickest smogs when I visited, and the University of North Carolina competed with Duke University, which had one of the strongest hematology programs in the country.

Then Dr. William Dameshek, the founding editor of *Blood: The American Journal of Hematology*, died on the operating table.

Henry Stratton, the publisher, called me. "Son,"—he always called me son—"Come to Boston next Friday. I'm giving a party for the members of the editorial board to introduce the new editor."

The party was in Fred Stohlman's home. Fred was the new editor. Cliff Gurney approached me during cocktails.

"Barth, how would you like to come to Kansas?"

"Kansas? What's in Kansas?"

"For one thing, I am."

"I didn't know that Cliff. I still have you in Princeton."

"Well, I am now the Chairman of Medicine at the University of Kansas. The American Cancer Society has created a new chair in clinical oncology at the university, and I wondered if you might be interested in taking that chair. It's the first of its kind in the country."

I was interested all right, and so was Nienke. Cliff arranged for a three-day visit and sent me a list of names of the senior staff he wanted me to meet. That was code for "We'd like to look you over before we decide to offer you the job." I went to the library of the New York Academy of Medicine and looked up what each name on the list had published in the last fifteen years. Three weeks later we took the plane to Kansas City, where Dr. Stan Friesen, the chairman of the search committee, met us at the airport. Our room in the Alameda Plaza Hotel overlooked the first shopping mall in the country. The next morning the wives of three staff members took Nienke under their wings and I made the rounds.

A pleasant chief of orthopedics eased me in for the day. He had no publications. Next came Dr. Jim Lowman, a pediatric hematologist. "I must apologize because I have the advantage over you," he said. "I have a copy of your CV and you know nothing about us."

"I liked your essay on iron deficiency anemia in children," I replied. "Did you consider whether folic acid deficiency played a role as well?"

We talked about that for the remainder of the half-hour. The other six interviewers that first day included Dr. Kermit Kranz, the Chairman of OB-GYN, who found it necessary to show off by chewing out a senior member of his staff on the phone. He grinned derisively when he put the phone down and said, "That's telling him, isn't it?" I had no comment. Kranz had no publications to speak off, but he did boast that he had screwed five stewardesses on the night that he and his wife's plane landed in Brussels. The evening, filled with cocktails and dinner, was at the home of the Chairman of Pediatrics, a Dr. Miller and his wife, whose father was the famed socialist Norman Thomas. She was delighted to talk with someone raised in Holland, a country with strong socialist overtones.

"How was your day?" I asked Nienke in the hotel.

"Very nice. They showed me around town and the suburbs where most of them live. And we had a nice lunch. I wouldn't mind living here." The shepherds had done a good job.

My first interview on the second day was with Professor Dante Scarpelli, the Chairman of Pathology. His secretary held his door open, and Dante came forward, but without looking at him I walked straight to an enormous aquarium against the wall across from his desk.

"So that's where you do your studies on cancer in fish?"

Was he ever surprised? Only then did we shake hands.

"How do you know that I study fish?" This second generation Italian could not stop talking about his fishes. He had done some excellent work in that little-known field. My last interview was with Stan Friesen, a gentleman and a Mennonite.

"Are you still operating on patients with Zollinger-Ellison syndrome?" I asked.

"So you know my interests too," he smiled. Word had gotten around. "What is your impression so far?"

"I have the feeling that some members on the staff do not like the word *cancer*."

"You are so right, especially in the Department of Medicine. The former chairman did not even want any cancer patients on his floors. He thought that young medical students should not be exposed to that dreadful disease."

"It's that bad?"

"It is also the main reason why the cancer society is giving the chair. Would you be interested in the job?"

"As long as the oncology division is in the Department of Medicine, I might be interested."

Stan drove Nienke and me to the airport. "I hope to see you again."

Two weeks later, he invited us for a second visit, which was a good sign. However, this time it would be for the annual meeting of the Kansas Division of the American Cancer Society. The meeting was in Hutchinson, Kansas, a prairie town where passing freight trains hoot all night. The division president welcomed the dignitaries on the dais, we received polite applause, and then it was time for the guest speaker of the evening to be introduced. "I'm sure you all know our distinguished senator Bob Dole, who will talk tonight about the government's support for cancer research. Senator Dole, ladies and gentlemen."

Dole stood, waved with his good arm, and moved behind the rostrum.

"Thank you Mr. President, it's nice to be amongst friends again. Coming home reminds me of a story that's close to my heart." While speaking, the senator removed a stack of cards from his pocket. The story received quite a laugh from the large audience, and Dole turned over the first card. "Let me tell you something I heard just before I left Washington."

The senator proceeded to tell one joke after another with the help of his cards. After twenty minutes or so, he finished the last card, put the stack back in his pocket, and said, "As far as support from the government for cancer research is concerned, I know nothing about it. Thank you." and he sat down to loud laughter and applause. He had earned his speaker's fee for the night.

Shortly after the second visit, I was offered the job as the first American Cancer Society Professor of Clinical Oncology, and we did not take long to make up our minds, even though it meant a drop in salary from $ 40,000 to $30,000. The challenge of creating an entirely new medical division in a school that thus far had neglected the cancer patient, was one of the main reasons why I was attracted to the job. I would start on July 1, 1970.

The rumor soon went around that I was going to Kansas and that it meant that I would have to leave the ALGB. Gordon Zubrod called.

"Barth, would you be interested in joining the Western Group?"

That group was headquartered in California and known for its low productivity. It took too long to complete the studies and the leadership was stale.

"Gordon, compared to the ALGB, that will be several notches down."

"That's why I called. You could bring some badly needed life to that group."

"I'll tell you how you can make it interesting. I have to become the group chairman."

"Barth, I can't do that. How about the Southeast Group? You know that Kansas is already a member of that group don't you?"

"Yes I do." The Southeast Group was an improvement over the Western Group, but still no ALGB. The group was mainly interested in chronic leukemia. "Let's see what the future will bring, Gordon."

A few days later I received a one-liner from Tom Frei, the chairman of the SWCCSG, the Southwest Cancer Chemotherapy Study Group. "Barth, don't forget that Kansas faces southwest. Tom."

I called Tom, and he invited me to the next group meeting in three weeks in San Antonio. The SWCCSG resembled the ALGB in large part. In addition to the leukemias, lymphomas, and multiple myeloma, the group also had a solid tumor committee chaired by Bob Talley of the Henry Ford Hospital in Detroit. Tom and I met in his hotel room.

"What will it take for you to join us, Barth?"

"The chairmanship of a study committee."

"Well, I can't give you lymphoma, because that's under Chuck Coltman. Alexanian has the myeloma, and J Freireich runs leukemia. That doesn't leave much."

"How about splitting off a solid tumor, Tom?"

"Like what?"

"Like breast. You let me have breast, and I'll join your group." I came straight from hematology and had never seen a patient with breast cancer. However, at that time there was no effective chemotherapy for metastatic breast cancer and this was where I could have some input.

"OK, it's a deal. How about the patients with leukemia, lymphoma and myeloma? Can you bring them in?"

"If you support my grant application, I'll swing it."

"I'm going to the University of Kansas," I said to Wasserman after I returned to New York City.

"What's in Kansas?"

"I'll be the first American Cancer Society Professor of Clinical Oncology."

He pursed his lips, nodded his head ever so slightly a couple of times, and said, "That's good. I like that. Are you staying with ALGB?"

"No, I made a deal with Tom Frei. I'll be his chairman for breast cancer."

"That'll be a switch. When do you start?"

"First day of July."

"Well I want you and Nienke to come to the apartment next Thursday evening for a little party."

Lou and Julia Wasserman invited the entire hematology staff to the party. Lou gave a little speech and presented us with a painting by the Hungarian painter Music. We gave them an antique statue of a Balinese dancer to express our gratitude for all they had done for us. After the guests left, we reminisced for a while in the study. On our way out, Lou suddenly opened the glass door of a display cabinet and handed me a magnificent ivory statue of a Japanese fisherman. "Here. Thank you." He turned and disappeared. It was as close to showing emotion I had ever seen him come. We had gone through some tough times together, but mostly through the best.

Immigrants know what leaving means. Nienke and I had left our families, our friends, and our country to live in another world and seek the adventure of a new future. We have experienced the hard reality of leaving, and we looked forward to a new life in Kansas, in the middle of the country. It was time for us to move on, taking fond memories of Lou and Julia Wasserman with us. By old Dutch custom, we have a birthday calendar that hangs in our bath room, the traditional spot for it. Lou's birthday has a place on July 11, and we always called him without fail. "I was waiting for your call," he would say. "I knew you would."

My new job was quite different from the one I had left, to say the least. In New York, I had three associates, four fellows, sixty-eight technicians, a secretarial staff, and a large budget. In Kansas, I did not even have a license to practice medicine. The Kansas Board of Regents insisted that the new professor of medicine sit for its examination. I did and passed without looking in a book. My office at KU was nine by eight feet and had no bookshelves. No budget, no associates, no fellows, and no technicians, but on the second day an attractive blond knocked on my always-open door.

"Come in, please. Who are you?"

"My name is Cherri Stadalman, and I want to be your secretary"

"Do you have experience as a medical secretary?"

"No, but I'm very good, and I know everything there is to know about computers. Besides that, my husband is a medical student."

"When can you start, Mrs. Stadalman?"

"I can start tomorrow, and, please, call me Cherri."

"Thank you. I'm curious, with all that experience, how old are you?"

"I'm twenty-three, and I'll never answer that question again."

It was the beginning of a great partnership.

Cliff stuck his head in. "I think you ought to pay Dr. Delp a visit."

"Who's he?"

"He was my predecessor for about twenty-five years. It's just a courtesy call."

Shirley, his secretary, escorted me to Dr. Delp's office. "I'll save you in thirty minutes," she whispered.

Delp was a small, lean man with a light brown complexion, gray hair and mustache. He wore a bolo tie with a silver clasp and green stone and a Western-style belt buckle with a green stone. His large, square office contained a desk and chair in one corner, an armchair in a second corner, and ten golfers' paces diagonal from it was a regular chair. On the bookshelves were only two books. He pointed to the third chair and sat in the armchair. No handshake, no word. He looked toward the window and turned a ring with a huge green stone around a finger on his left hand. Around and around went the ring, and I was damned if I was going to say the first word. About ten minutes later his head turned, and he took his time looking me over. Then it was back to the window.

"So you're the one who is going to teach about cancer to my students?" It was more like a statement than a question, and I remained silent. "They are too young, and they have plenty to learn about good diseases."

I had to admit, but did not say, that cancer is not a good disease to have.

"In my time I didn't want those patients on my floors and it is a damn mistake to start now." He went back to turning the ring. I still had not said a word.

One of the two books was the Physician's Desk Reference and the other was about physical diagnosis. Delp's name and that of another physician were on the cover.

"May I ask who the other doctor is on that book?" There was no sense talking about oncology with the man. He was likely not to know what the word meant.

"That is Professor Ralph Major. You have heard of him, of course."

"No sir, I have not." Big mistake.

"You damn well ought to have." Agitated, he got up and pointed to the door. I had said sixteen words, and there was no need for Shirley to save me.

"Who is Ralph Major?" I asked Gurney during lunch.

"He was the chairman before Delp. He had a severe stroke several months ago and has been in the hospital ever since. He is unconscious, but Delp visits him every day."

"Have you read his book?"

"No, but he thinks that it is the bible of physical diagnosis. Every student was expected to buy a copy while he was chairman."

"Nice little income. You, uh...stopped that practice I presume?"

Cliff smiled and let it drop.

This new professor of clinical oncology started without students, with borrowed clinic time, and with no referrals. I had clinic twice a week and waited three weeks before the first patient showed, but she did not have cancer. However, I did have a convenient parking place. The administrative buildings surrounded a square inner court used for parking by about fifteen important people and was guarded by an officer with a friendly face. The first morning on the job I drove into the court, and the guard waved a no-no finger at me. He had a nametag, and I got out.

"Good morning, Mr. Taylor. I am the new cancer doctor, and I need a parking place."

"Cancer you say? My wife had a breast taken off two years ago. She had cancer."

"Well she has a good chance that she is cured, but if there's any trouble, you just call me."

"Let me see now...where can I fit you in? How about right here?"

It was the second space from the main entrance, next to the one for the dean.

"Thank you, Mr. Taylor. I won't forget that."

I was invited to conduct a CPC during the second month at KU. The monthly Clinical Pathological Conference was *the* conference in every medical school and large hospital in the country. The pathologist selected an interesting patient, wrote a one or two page abstract of the case, and invited a guest speaker or member of the staff to discuss the case and venture a diagnosis. The pathologists had the last word, and they loved to fool the speaker.

The auditorium was packed, as is usual for a CPC. The senior staff sat in the first row, Scarpelli next to Gurney. I took the audience through the abstract, asked the radiologist to discuss the X-rays, and was surprised when he showed only X-rays of the chest. He described the large tumor close to the right side of the heart and sat down. That did not leave me with much to make a diagnosis. However, I did remember old Professor Snapper's advice: "Always keep your eye on the pathologist. When he is happy you are discussing the wrong diagnosis."

"It is obvious to all of you that we are dealing with a tumor in the chest and the first diagnosis that comes to mind is, of course, lung cancer."

Dante Scarpelli was happy.

I proceeded to discuss the presentation of lung cancer. "But I do not believe that this patient had lung cancer."

Dante sat upright.

"Could she have a lymphoma such as Hodgkin's disease?"

Dante relaxed.

I filled time talking about lymphoma and mentioned a few other possibilities. Dante remained relaxed.

"A few things are troubling me about this case. Only X-rays of the chest were presented and no follow-up of the patient's condition was given. Cancer progresses during the course of the disease, and I find it strange that no other X-rays were taken." Did I see Dante stiffen a bit? "And why does the abstract only cover one admission?" Dante and the other pathologists felt the need to move about in their seats. "Could it be that this patient did not have cancer?"

Dr. Scarpelli sat upright, and I knew I had him.

"I think that we're dealing with a pseudo lymphoma."

Dante looked at Gurney with a shrug of his shoulders. I discussed the fascinating topic of pseudo lymphoma and ended with, "That is my diagnosis."

"You tried to fool me, didn't you?" I said to Scarpelli after the conference. He laughed.

"How were you so sure?" he asked.

"That'll remain my secret."

In-house consultations and referrals to the clinic picked up after that CPC. A tall gentleman knocked on my door. "Doctor Hoogstraten? I am Doctor Wilson, and I'd like to turn a patient over to you. It's a man I operated on eight years ago for a large tumor in his abdomen.

"What did the biopsy show?"

"According to the pathologist it was a very malignant tumor."

"And that was eight years ago?" This had the makings of an unlikely story.

"It sounds impossible doesn't it, but that's what happened. I gave him a prescription and told him to go fishing."

"You're doing so well, why send him to me?"

"Well, I've been a surgeon for thirty-two years and it's time to quit. I have a small farm near Newton, a few ponds stocked with bass, and I am going fishing and do a little hunting."

Doctor Wilson was a contented man on his way to a well-deserved retirement.

Chuck came to my clinic a week later. He was a bear of a man, sixty-three years old, and he appeared to be in perfect health. I examined him and found nothing wrong.

"What did Dr. Wilson tell you?" I asked.

"He said that I had a bad tumor, cancer you know, and that he couldn't remove it."

"Did he do anything else?"

"He gave me a pill to take." Chuck did not volunteer much.

"So what next? What happened to the swelling?"

"It went away," he said.

"You mean you had a large swelling that you could feel and it just went away?"

"Yes. Took a few months, but it all disappeared."

"What about the pills? How long did you take those?"

"Still take 'em doc—one every day."

"Did you bring them with you? Can I see one?"

Chuck showed me an old bottle with the pills. Cytoxan, 25 mg tablets they were.

I needed more information about this puzzling case, and gave him an appointment for one month. The operating note described a football-sized tumor that had infiltrated into the surrounding tissue. The pathology report was that of a highly undifferentiated cancer. I sat down with the pathologist at the microscope and there was indeed a wild cancer with numerous dividing cells.

"Would you mind if I send the slides and the block to AFIP?" I asked the pathologist.

"No, go right ahead."

I sent the slides and the tissue block from which the slides had been made to a friend at the Armed Forces Institute for Pathology in Washington and three weeks later his report can back. "A highly undifferentiated malignant tumor." The patient should have died shortly after his surgery.

"Chuck you are one lucky man," I said when he saw me.

"Yes I am."

"Now about the Cytoxan pills. You can stop taking them."

"Oh no doctor. That pill is my crutch. I'll take one for the rest of my life."

I could not argue with success and saw Chuck every six months for the next eleven years, when he was still going strong. He certainly was a medical miracle.

I was still working alone when Ron Stephens came to see me. He was the senior fellow in hematology. "I would like to be an oncology fellow with you."

"Where were you born, Ron?"

"In Wichita."

"Went to school in Wichita?"

"Yes sir."

"KU medical school and residency?"

"Yes."

"So you can't teach me anything new can you? No new procedure?"

"No sir, not really."

"Tell you what, Ron. You get out of here for a year, and when you come back I'll consider you."

Ron was determined. "Can you recommend a place?"

"I want you to go to the NCI for a year. Don't worry; I'll do the calling if you are serious about becoming an oncologist."

Ron was serious, and I called the NCI. He took his wife and two daughters to Bethesda, Maryland, and was a clinical associate at the NCI for a year.

"Learned anything I don't already know?" I asked when he showed up again.

"I can do spleen punctures."

Ron not only became my first fellow in Kansas, he succeeded me. He specialized in genitourinary tumors, was appointed chairman of an NIH study section and above all he was the best teacher I had ever encountered. Ron's presence freed up time for me, enough to pay attention to the breast cancer committee. A new drug, Adriamycin, had just completed the Phase I evaluation, and I selected it for an extensive evaluation in metastatic cancer of the breast. It soon proved to be very active and for our next study we compared Adriamycin with combination chemotherapy of three drugs. Both studies were completed in record time and published in 1975–1976.

Tom Frei called from Houston. "Barth, you may have heard that I am leaving the MD Anderson Hospital and the SWCCSG. I'm calling to ask your support for—"

"Tom, if you're asking me to vote for Freireich as the next group chairman, I can't do that."

"I understand, but J is a good friend, and I had to ask."

"I just don't think that he'll be a good leader, Tom."

The group was to meet the next week, and the election was on the agenda. However, Tom unexpectedly announced that he would stay on as chairman for another four months and divide his time between Houston and Boston. The reason was obvious: His man did not have the votes. Three candidates besides J Freireich had turned up, and MD Anderson's president, Dr. R. Lee Clark, went to work to keep the chairmanship at Anderson. The NCI grant for the group headquarters brought quite a sizeable sum of money to the institution in the form of indirect costs, and the SWCCSG brought esteem to MD Anderson.

Dr. De Bakey at Baylor convinced Monty Lane that it was best for all concerned if he withdrew his candidacy. Bill Levin of the University of Texas Medical Branch in Galveston had served as group chairman from 1963 to 1967 before Tom took over. Bill was promoted to president of that branch, which prevented him from being group chairman. Rumor had it that Chuck Coltman of the Lackland Air Force Base was promised the directorship of the Department of Medicine at MD Anderson after he completed his twenty years of service. The road was now clear for the only remaining candidate, Freireich.

New Orleans was the scene of the 1972 election. The group met for its normal morning schedule, and around eleven o'clock I went to the men's room. I turned around to wash my hands and was confronted by three members: Levin, Lane and Arthur Haut of the University of Arkansas.

"Barth, we would like you to run for the chairmanship," said Arthur.

He might as well have knocked me down.

"Wait a minute; I've been in the group only a year and a half. Can't you find someone else?"

"We have considered that, and it comes down to you," Monty said.

"Gentlemen, I owe a large part of my career to the NCI and will not do anything without its approval."

Bill Levin picked up a phone, dialed a number, listened, and handed it to me. A voice said, "It's OK with us, Doctor Hoogstraten." Click.

Tom opened the meeting after lunch with, "The meeting will come to order for the election of the new group chairman. There is only one candidate, and I call for a show of hands in unanimous support for Dr. J Freireich."

Arthur Haut rose from the back rows. "Mr. Chairman, I nominate Dr. Barth Hoogstraten."

It took poor Tom completely by surprise. The room was silent, waiting. Someone shouted that the nomination needed a second.

"I second the nomination," Monty Lane said dryly.

Tom called for a recess. "The principal investigators will meet in the next room."

I took Cherri and our nurse to the coffee shop to calm them down. An hour later the meeting reconvened.

"The nomination of Dr. Hoogstraten appears to be in order, and we will proceed with the election," Tom said. "Only principal investigators can vote."

Ten minutes later the ballots were counted, and Tom announced the results. "Dr. Freireich fifteen votes, Dr. Hoogstraten sixteen votes."

Cherri, sitting next to me, pinched me hard in my side.

"There will be a fifteen-minute recess," Tom shouted over the noisy crowd.

I got up and walked to Tom, who was on his way out to the airport.

"Congratulations Barth," he said. "I have to run, but I'll write you from Boston."

Freireich came storming at me. "You're finished," he fumed. "We'll see to it that you'll never get another grant. You're a nothing. We'll squash you like an ant and ship you back to New York where you came from." He was one of those individuals who could not control himself once he gets going, and he was beyond being angry, menacing me that way. When his stabbing finger came too close to my chest I slapped his hand away. He had just suffered his second defeat. When Tom left the NCI for MD Anderson in 1963, Jim Holland had beaten Freireich in the election for the chairmanship of the ALGB. This autocratic man, who looked down on his colleagues, was not smart enough to realize that his peers would never elect him.

A serious Ray Alexanian, also from MD Anderson, came over after J disappeared. "Barth, the best advice I can give you is that you go straight from here to Houston and explain what happened to R. Lee Clark."

"I don't see what he has to do with this, Ray."

"Oh a lot. You really should go and see him." Ray meant well, but I did not go.

I called the meeting back to order, said the customary words of thanks and promises and stepped away from the podium so that the committee chairmen could go on with their work. That evening I heard a rumor that group statistician Ed Gehan was going to challenge the outcome of the vote.

I opened the meeting at 8:30 AM, and Ed got up, but I was one step ahead of him.

"I understand that there is a question about the legality of yesterday's vote. I appoint Drs. Vietti, Coltman, and Haut to investigate the matter and report back to the chair. In the meantime, the meeting will continue." Two hours later Chuck Coltman reported that the vote was legal and would stand. At the end of the meeting, I also appointed an ad hoc committee to draft a new constitution and bylaws for the group. Chuck Coltman represented the adult division, Don Fernbach of Baylor the pediatric division, Ed Gehan for the statistical side, and Cherri Stadelman would act as secretary.

Tom Frei was now the new physician-in-chief of the Children's Cancer Research Foundation in Boston. He wrote, "Excepting J, I think you are overwhelmingly the best choice the group could have made, and I am indeed proud to have been succeeded by you." It was the kind of support I more than welcomed for the job ahead.

Two weeks later I visited the group headquarters in Houston. Group Administrator Dorothy Abernathy escorted me to a small conference room. "I look forward working with you," she volunteered.

Gehan, two other statisticians, and Group Secretary Dr. Jeffrey Gottlieb joined us. Jeff was another former NCI man. He was a pediatrician by training, but after he joined Tom Frei, he converted to the study of cancer in adults. "I'll show you around the administrative offices later," he said.

"I don't think that'll be necessary Jeff; I'm moving them to Kansas City."

The announcement floored them.

"It'll be easier to keep them here, and you can come visit us," Abernathy said.

"No Dorothy, they are going to Kansas. By the way, Cherri Stadelman will be the new Group Administrator." Abernathy did not say another word.

"Also, I am changing the name of the group. From now on it will be called the Southwest Oncology Group."

Another moment of silence, broken by Gehan. "What will people call it, SOG or SWOG?" he asked rather sarcastically.

"SWOG will do fine Ed, and there will be other changes. We will become a multidisciplinary group. I am inviting the surgeons, radiation therapists, pathologists, and gynecologists to join the group; therefore the acronym SWCCSG is no longer appropriate—and another thing: I am not pleased with the quality of the patient records. We are going to set a higher standard from now on. For the time being all records will have to come to Kansas first."

I knew that this last item would meet a lot of resistance, and I was not disappointed.

"That will create an unnecessary delay," Jeff said.

"I realize that, but unless you can come up with a better idea, I'll insist."

Cherri and I had already considered another way of handling it, but I wanted Ed Gehan to come up with it.

"The records can still come here and we will immediately send you a copy," he said. "Then we can work on the analyses while you check the quality."

I had hoped that he would suggest that, and we agreed.

"By the way Jeff, I would very much like you to stay on as group secretary."

He was pleased.

Back home, Cherri and I made plans for the new group, and I went to see the new chairman of medicine, Dr. Norton Greenberger. Cliff Gurney had left to become dean of the University of Chicago Medical School. Nortie was delighted when I told him about SWOG and the changes that had taken place. I asked for his support, which he gladly gave. "Having the group headquarters here is a feather in the cap of KU," he said. Of course, he did not have the space to house the headquarters and neither did the dean. Cherri came up with a brilliant idea. She called the recently opened Rosedale Bank on nearby Rainbow Boulevard and asked whether there was space for rent. There was, and the bank director was pleased to give us the entire basement for a very reasonable price. She estimated that we would need at least six secretaries or clerks, furniture, typewriters, computers, a copying machine, and numerous supplies. My initial grant request was big, but approved without trouble and in record time.

"Are you ready for a liquid lunch?" Cherri asked one day.

I had no idea what she had in mind, but went along anyway. The next group meeting would take place in four weeks, and we needed to do some planning. We also had not heard anything from the ad hoc committee for the bylaws, and I began to smell a rat. The alcohol stimulated our brain cells and out came many ideas for her to remind me of several weeks or months later. Cherri never wrote anything down; her brain was a steel trap, and she remembered everything. I never ceased to be amazed when she reminded me of something we had brought up six or even eight months before.

"One of the pharmaceutical companies has offered to pay for a reception if it's all right with you," she said.

I had no objection. I had informed the principal investigators (PIs) of the group of my plan to convert SWOG from a simple chemotherapy group into a multidisciplinary one and urged them to bring a surgeon, radiotherapist, and pathologist to the meeting in San Antonio. A reception was ideal for the introductions.

In my hotel room at 11:00 AM, Coltman, Fernbach, and Gehan sat down and presented me with their draft of the new bylaws. All I needed to see was the organizational chart. There was to be an adult division with a chairperson, a pediatric division with a chairperson, and a statistical office with Gehan in the center. The position of group chairman was eliminated, and specialties other than medical oncology were not included.

"Thank you gentlemen, that'll be all."

They looked at each other. "Aren't you going to comment?" Fernbach asked.

"No."

Coltman sat next to me at lunch. "You're very quiet."

"Chuck, you don't think for a minute that I'm going to take this laying down do you?"

He smiled. "I don't expect you to."

"By the way, who acted as secretary for this?"

"Dorothy Abernathy."

After lunch, I announced that I had received a draft of the bylaws and we would consider the draft during the next meeting. I then asked the PIs and their guest to meet with me in another hall.

"Thank you all for coming on such short notice. Your PI has informed you of my plan to convert SWOG into a multidisciplinary group, and I'd like to hear your thoughts about it."

For the next twenty minutes I answered questions.

"I'd now like each specialty to split off and come up with a plan for how you will best fit into the multidisciplinary format. I'll circulate to answer questions."

I was amazed by how well the idea of integrated participation in the group studies was received. With one exception, I asked each specialty to select a leader. The exception was for pathology, for which I recommended Dr. Robert McDivitt from Utah. I had read some of his articles on breast cancer and had serendipitously met him in the elevator the night before. We were off to a good start.

"Forget that draft of the bylaws," I told Cherri when we were back in Kansas. "We'll write our own draft."

The drafters had made a mistake when they omitted the other specialties from their draft. I had set the multidisciplinary approach to cancer research in motion, and both PIs and the NCI were in favor of it. I had also encouraged each PI to amend his or her grant request to include funding for a surgeon, pathologist, and radiotherapist and invited Dr. Palmer Saunders, the NCI official responsible for the funding of the cooperative group program, to the next Group meeting. One month before the meeting Cherri sent a copy of the two drafts for the constitution and bylaws to each PI.

The meeting took place in Houston and Cherri had organized a cocktail party for all members for the first evening. Saunders attended, but only one PI showed up.

"Where are the PIs?" I asked Cherri, who raised her shoulders in response.

It did not take long to find out. They were at a reception in J Freireich's home to which I had not been invited. Was he by chance trying to influence the vote for the bylaws? After lunch the second day, I introduced Palmer Saunders, who, with some help from me, knew very well what was going on. He congratulated the group on taking the important step of inviting the other disciplines to participate in our studies. He wished us well and promised his support. The PIs listened carefully, especially when he mentioned support.

"We will now vote by institution on the proposed drafts for a new constitution and bylaws for the group," I announced. "We'll take the draft marked A
first. All PIs in favor of that draft raise your hands. Cherri, please count them."

"Twenty-seven," she said.

"All those opposed?"

"Four votes."

"Thank you Cherri. Well, with that count there doesn't seem to be a need for
another vote, and unless I hear an objection draft A is adopted."

It was our draft. The presence of Palmer Saunders undoubtedly had some
influence on the vote, but so did Freireich's miscalculation. Several PIs were
angry when they had noticed that I was not at his house the evening before.
"That really pissed us off," was the general sentiment.

The new SWOG was ready to grow. It had four new standing committees for
surgery, pathology, radiotherapy, and immunology-immunotherapy. We welcomed the University of Arizona into our ranks, and when Chuck Coltman
retired from the Air Force and started an oncology program at the University of
Texas at San Antonio, he too continued as an important member.

Rose Ruth Ellison, the president-elect of the American Society of Clinical
Oncology (ASCO) asked me to chair its program committee and the clinical program of the American Association for Cancer Research (AACR) for the 1976
meetings. That included appointing the session chairmen. It was customary for
the program chairman to chair one of the main sessions, and I wanted Jeff Gottlieb to chair the session with me. However, I did not know whether he would be
physically able to do it. Jeff had received massive doses of chemotherapy in a last
attempt to get a remission for his far-advanced cancer. His blood counts were
exceedingly low, so low that infection had to be avoided at all costs. He was con-
fined to a completely enclosed plastic tent—called a Life Island—for total steril-
ity. Jeff knew the score. I went to see him in Houston.

"I'd like you to co-chair the main session at ASCO with me, Jeff."

"That'll be an honor." He was short of breath.

"You think you can swing it?"

He weakly smile behind the plastic. "That depends how this chemo works
out. I can't promise you, Barth, but if at all possible I'll be there."

Jeff came to San Diego the day before the session. The next morning he went
to a nearby hospital to have fluid removed from his chest. In the afternoon he
took his place next to me and—with his beautiful, sonorous voice—called the
session to order. More fluid was removed before he flew back to Houston the

next day, and he went straight to the hospital from the plane. Jeff died a few weeks later.

One of the most important impacts effects of the cooperative group program was the funding to train oncology fellows in the participating hospitals. After completing their fellowship many of them went out into the community to treat cancer patients. However, they did not want to lose contact with the groups and asked whether they could enter their patients on the protocol studies. Unfortunately, the chairmen did not have the funds to do this, and in 1974–1975 a cry went up in the communities to ask Congress for the funds. Congress responded with an allocation of five million dollars, and the NCI appointed Dr. Diane Fink of the then-defunct Western VA Group to run this new outreach program. Jim Holland, John Durant of the Southeast Group, and I asked for a meeting with Dr. Richard Rauscher, the new NCI director. The three of us met the night before, and, after some discussion, we agreed to ask for two million dollars.

"Dick, we think that the groups are in the best position to lend a hand to that new outreach program," Jim said, opening the discussion. "We trained the fellows who are now out there in the community, and we can provide them with the drugs and the protocols."

"Diane needs help to get her program started, and she'll welcome us with open arms," I said.

"She'll be happy to use part of the five million dollars for that purpose," John added.

Rauscher, a virologist with a virus named after him, recognized the logic of letting the groups play a role in the new outreach program, and he called Diane to his office.

"You know these gentlemen, I'm sure."

"I haven't met Dr. Durant before, but I know Dr. Holland and have talked with Barth a few times," Diane said, smiling.

"They think that the groups can help you start your program, but they need some money to do this. What are your thoughts about that?"

Diane was asked to run a new program on short notice, and she needed all the help she could get. "It is the best idea I've heard thus far."

"But are you willing to pay for it?" I asked. "It'll increase our work load in the operations office and in statistics considerably."

"How about two million, Diane?" Jim asked.

Diane looked at Dick, who nodded approvingly, and she agreed.

"OK, that's settled. I leave it to you to work out the details. Thank you for coming." Rauscher ended the meeting. With that, the groups entered into an outreach program, soon to be called the Cooperative Group Outreach Program, or CGOP.

16

A CALL FROM THE STATE DEPARTMENT

"The State Department is on the line," my secretary said in an excited voice.

I picked up my phone.

"Doctor Hoogstraten, this is the Egyptian desk. Just a moment for Ambassador Eilts please."

I could hear her in the background telling someone that I was on the line.

Ambassador Hermann Eilts was a man of few words. "Doctor, I would like you to come to Cairo to evaluate the Egyptian National Cancer Institute."

"Is there a specific reason why I should go, Mr. Ambassador?"

"Yes, they would like to become a member of your group, and I understand that you have to approve all requests for membership."

"Mr. Ambassador, I'll come, but only if my administrator can accompany me." Cherri should look into the administrative setup of the institute.

"That's fine with me. The desk here and Professor Elsebai of the institute will make all the arrangements. Thank you doctor."

It turned out that during World War II, the United States had frozen all Egyptian funds. While President Nasser leaned heavily toward Communist Russia, our government refused to release these funds. However, on September 28, 1970, Nasser died of a heart attack, and Anwar al-Sadat became the new president. He quickly threw off the heavy yoke Moscow had placed on Egypt in return for selling some outdated weapons and became friendly to the United States. Sadat visited the US, charmed the politicians, and reminded President Nixon of the funds. Nixon sent Kissinger to Cairo where he was wined, dined, and shown the sights. During the course of his visit, he and his Egyptian counterpart agreed that the first funds would be used for health issues.

When our TWA plane landed at the airport in Heliopolis, Egypt, the door swung open and the first class stewardess requested that the passengers remain seated. A gentleman entered and said something to the stewardess, who pointed me out to him.

"Professor Hoogstraten, I represent the United States Embassy. Welcome to Egypt, sir. Your passport, please? Will you follow me?"

I handed him my passport and followed after him. At the foot of the stairs he introduced me to Drs. Mohammed Mansour and Nazli Gad El-Mawla. They escorted me to the VIP reception room and handed me the first of thousands of soft drinks and tea. Cherri and her husband entered ten minutes later, and we left in three cars to go to the Meridian Hotel without having gone through immigration or customs. My luggage was already in my room when I entered. Dr. Mansour (everybody called him Mo) turned out to be the chief surgeon of the Egyptian National Police, and he was responsible for our smooth entry into Egypt.

That evening Dr. Elsebai entertained us for dinner at the Sheraton Hotel, where the roof of the restaurant opened to the stars in the sky and the wife of the manager performed an exquisite belly dance. She hardly moved at all, just a delicate rippling of her abdominal muscles, slow, fast, and faster with the music. Elsebai was a man of the world in his sixties who was bald, sunburned, soft spoken, and had a heavyset body and jaws and a genuine laugh. He had a commanding presence and was an object of admiration and devotion. Inevitably some members of the staff could barely suppress their envy and their eagerness to displace him.

In the morning we were introduced to the staff of the cancer institute. Cherri disappeared for the rest of the day into administration, and I listened to presentations in fairly good English by serious staff members. The only research worth mention was conducted by Professor El-Bolkainy of the pathology department and by Dr. Ghoneim, a professor of urology at Mansoura University. The rest of the research was basic and long ago outdated, but presented with such intense sincerity that I felt obliged to pay close attention. They showed me their laboratories and pointed with pride to the few instruments, and again I paid attention, smiled, complimented, and discussed them. The library contained some outdated textbooks and years-old issues of a few journals; most shelves were empty.

The hospital rooms were clean enough, but the little space between the narrow beds left no room for furniture. The beds had thin mattresses covered with clean sheets that had once been white. Silent faces of sick men and women stared at us. Hollow cheeks and wide-open eyes deep in their sockets signaled the imminent death of some. Family members prepared meals for the patients in the hallways. On the pediatric floor the children slept two or three to a bed, feet to head. Clinic patients crowded the suffocating waiting rooms and overflowed into a courtyard and onto the streets. There were ugly wounds barely covered with pieces of cloth and large tumors disfiguring necks and faces. Patients on home-made stretchers waiting in the heat of the midday sun while sons and daughters waved flies away. The silence struck me most of all.

That evening Cherri and her husband were sick as dogs with vomiting and diarrhea. Fortunately I was immunized to the hazards of food and drink during my three years in Indonesia and suffered no ill effects. Dr. Gad El-Mawla, who soon became Nazli, and Dr. Hassan Awwad, the chairman of the radiotherapy department with the one cobalt machine donated by Phillips of Holland and one 250 KV machine, treated me to "The City of Lights." Nazli drove us to the town of Giza, passed a wide expanse of thousands of chairs, and stopped at the first row. Only our car was permitted this convenience, the other visitors walked from a distant parking place.

Nazli showed me my chair and proudly said, "You sit where two months ago Mr. Kissinger sat." I feigned importance for her benefit and enjoyed a beautiful show of music and lights playing on the pyramids and the Sphinx. The next morning Dr. Elsebai painted a glum picture. "Egypt has gone backwards since the beginning of World War II. There was little or nothing we could do during the war because the English did not trust us. Maybe with good reason," he said with a pause and a little smile. "Then King Farouk became a playboy and gambled our reserves away in Monte Carlo. Nasser brought the Russians in after the United States refused to pay for the construction of the Aswan Dam, which is a mistake anyway, and the West put a stop to our exports. We have to start at the bottom." He threw up his hands, "Now you know it all, Barth."

"May I ask why cancer was chosen as the first project? I would have thought that the money would be better spent on bandages, antibiotics, and new surgical instruments."

He smiled. "You are right, of course, but then you cannot measure results, and our new American friends want to see the results." He shrugged his massive shoulders and smiled, "And maybe I pushed a little."

I laughed. "I understand; just a little."

With what I had seen during those two days, I had already decided to approve the request. These doctors needed help badly, and it had to start somewhere. Why not with this cancer institute?

"Dr. Elsebai—"

His hand stopped me. "Ismail, please."

"All right Ismail, if I approve the request, I must make one thing perfectly clear. I'll decide who will attend the SWOG meetings. I will not accept a bunch of surgeons who are eager for a free trip to the US and not going to contribute to the group."

He was very serious. "The American embassy must approve all travel, but tell me what you want, and I'll see what I can do."

"To begin with, I want you at all meetings. Dr. Awwad for radiotherapy, Dr. Gad El-Mawla because she is the only medical oncologist, and Dr. El-Bolkainy for pathology."

"Consider it done. What else do you need from me?"

"I want the children, especially those with leukemia. But you do not have a pediatric oncologist on your staff."

"Not to worry. A young doctor is finishing her hematology training in Paris, and I will give her an appointment as a pediatric oncologist." He had to overcome a lot of resistance from the all-male staff when he had appointed Nazli, and adding one more woman would only increase his reputation as a maverick.

The Board of SWOG accepted Egypt as a new member and Nazli worked wonders with one nurse and the enthusiastic support of the two fellows assigned to her by Elsebai. My stipulation that I would decide who would attend the group meetings turned out to be a fortunate one. However, a year later Elsebai reached the mandatory retirement age for deans of the University of Cairo and under his successor, Dr. Shahbander, a surgeon of Iraqi descent, a squabble erupted between the surgeons as to who would visit the US next. Shahbander knocked Dr. El-Bolkainy and the pediatrician off the list, added himself and two surgeons, and the embassy approved the list. I refused to accept the joyriders.

"The State Department is on the line again," my secretary announced.

"Just a moment for the Egyptian desk," a voice said, then a second voice, "Just a moment for Ambassador Eilts."

"Doctor, you are interfering with State Department business." Eilts sounded like a man who was used to getting his way.

"And you, Mr. Ambassador, are interfering with SWOG business."

There was a moment of silence at the other end before Eilts came back. "Then it looks like a stand-off doctor. What do you suggest?"

"Sir, my bylaws require one surgeon, the medical and pediatric oncologists, the radiotherapist, and the pathologist to attend the group meetings. I do not care much who the surgeon is, but I doubt that the new dean will step aside. That makes five people."

Eilts of course did not know that there was nothing in the SWOG bylaws about attendance to the group meetings.

"Doctor, I have to keep the peace with those people. What if I approve one extra traveler? Would that be OK with you?"

"That would be an excellent solution, Mr. Ambassador."

Years later I read somewhere that Kissinger considered Eilts as one of the United States' best ambassadors. I think I understood, in part, why.

17

EXTRACURRICULAR ACTIVITIES

Chairing SWOG was time consuming, and so were the extraneous functions. The NCI had recently created a program to bring basic science research and clinical research closer together. The aim was speedy transfer of new laboratory findings into the clinic. To create interest, the NCI waved a large carrot in the form of long-term funding for what were to be called Designated Cancer Centers. Several universities responded, and the NIH created a cancer center support grant review committee to evaluate the applications. I was a member of that body.

It was interesting work because it gave me an opportunity see how other medical schools approached cancer research and education. Two benefits immediately became evident: The basic scientists were intrigued to see cancer patients and be taking new ideas back to their laboratories; the clinicians learned to think more like basic scientists. The secretary of the review committee and his staff assisted the universities in writing the applications and appointed teams of scientists to visit each university. These site visit teams were chaired by a member of the committee, assisted by at least one or two other members and between ten and twelve scientists from around the country. It was true peer review. Members of the committee met every three or four months at the NIH to discuss the reports of the site visits and to make a final judgment.

I chaired the visits of some major institutions such as the Mayo Clinic and Yale University. At the start of each visit, I tried to relax both the members of the team and the hosts and was fortunate when Yale offered me an ideal opening. We met in the imposing boardroom, with its aged green-leather chairs, enormous conference table, and portraits of past-presidents looking down from the walls. As was customary, the president of Yale gave a welcoming speech to which I responded.

"Sir, I have the distinct impression that you keep your meetings short."

Somewhat puzzled, he said, "As a matter of fact I do, but how do you know?"

"Well, I have to sit here for three days and this is a most uncomfortable chair. I keep sliding forward and am in danger of landing on the floor."

"You too?" he laughed, as did the others.

Some twenty-five years later, I had an occasion to write the current president, Dr. Levin, and reminded him of the chair. "It is still there," he responded, "and you just reminded me to look for a secondhand one."

Not every welcoming speech was pleasant. The provost of a less renowned university gave the shortest speech, which he started with, "As far as I am concerned this idea of a cancer center has split the whole goddamn faculty in half."

After he finished, I called for a short executive session. "I know what you are all thinking—shall we leave now or later? It will have to be later. We have to hear what the faculty has to say; however, I doubt that we'll need more than a day and a half." We not surprisingly disapproved that grant application.

The staff of the proposed cancer centers always made presentations of their research to the site visitors, who would ask questions afterwards. That sometimes led to heated exchanges, so much so that one time I had to intervene by cutting off a site visitor. During the coffee break, I reminded the site visitors that we were guests and were there to listen and not impose our opinions on the hosts.

With millions riding on each grant application, the members of the host team were often somewhat anxious. While one young assistant professor presented her research, I noticed that she became pale and broke out in a sweat. I was about to say something nice to her, when she swayed left, right, and I yelled, "Catch her!" The poor woman was out cold for a while. When she came to and had a sip of water, she courageously continued her presentation. Needless to say that dedication persuaded us to vote in favor of her research project.

After Gordon Zubrod and Nat Berlin retired from the NCI and became directors of cancer centers in Miami and Chicago, respectively, they too joined the Cancer Center Review Committee. Nat chaired the visit to San Francisco where several universities and medical centers applied for funding of a cancer center "without walls," meaning neither Stanford nor the University of California nor the University of San Francisco was going to be *the* center. Instead it was going to be the Northern California Cancer Program with Dr. Stephen K. Carter, the leader at the NCI of the chemotherapy trials program, as director. However, Steve was not at the site visit and neither had he written the grant request. Leading scientists from the three institutions, people we all regarded as our peers, made the presentations of the research projects, and when it was over we were all impressed.

"Shall we call for a vote to approve the application?" Nat said as he opened our executive session. This was his first site visit and the secretary had mistakenly made him the chairman. It takes the experience of two or more visits before one can be an effective chairman.

"Why don't we discuss it first," someone said.

"What's there to discuss? They presented superb research."

Nat had spent most of his career at the NCI, and he was new to the academia.

"For one thing, this is not a cancer center grant; it is a program," I said. "And I seriously doubt that these people can work together."

The other site visitors joined in by pointing out several other problems, and it became clear that we could not wholeheartedly support the application. However, some of us knew that Steve had run into trouble at the NCI and needed a job.

"I recommend that we fund the salary of Dr. Carter as the director of the program and that we give him an assistant and a secretary. Let's give him a year or two and see whether he can pull it together." My proposal carried, and, at least temporarily, we saved the NCI several millions.

"I certainly learned quickly," Nat remarked after he adjourned the session. Eighteen months later Steve had created a successful outreach program in Northern California without the three universities contributing a penny.

Gordon Zubrod also learned quickly during his first site visit. On the last day he had a five o'clock plane back to Miami, and before we went into executive session he said to me, "I better call the airline and change to a later plane."

"Gordon, why don't you ask for an earlier plane? This won't take long."

He got on a three-forty plane. On the way to our next site visit a fellow member of the review committee and I sat next to each other in the plane. We were both in our last year.

"Have you any idea how much we're going to recommend?" he asked.

"I think so."

"Tell you what. Why don't we each write down a figure and at the end of the visit we'll see how close we came," he suggested.

The application was for several million and, as we had anticipated, it was approved. When we compared figures afterwards, we were only two thousand apart. We were ready to retire. I had learned a lot over the years and believe that we had contributed to the cancer centers program.

The International Union Against Cancer, headquartered in Geneva, is supported by the cancer organizations of every country. In 1984, the Union began a new project designated Current Treatment of Cancer. They invited as committee members Professor Julian Bloom of the Royal Marsden Hospital in London, Mr.

Ian Burn of the British Association of Surgical Oncology, Professor Folke Edsmyr of the Karolinska Sjukhuset in Stockholm, Professor Roberto Estevez of Buenos Aires, Dr. Joseph Fortner of Memorial Sloan-Kettering Cancer Center in New York City, and myself. Professor Ismail Elsebai of Egypt chaired the committee. We decided to publish a series of books on the latest cancer therapies aimed at developing and underdeveloped countries.

We tackled lung cancer first, because the people of the world continued to be heavy smokers. I edited the resultant book, but rather than select authors from many countries, we concentrated on the approach to the diagnosis and treatment of lung cancer in three outstanding institutions, the Brompton Hospital in London, the Finsen Institute in Copenhagen and the Memorial Sloan-Kettering Cancer Center in New York City. By limiting ourselves to these three institutions, we wanted to stress the importance of a team approach to cancer.

I edited a book called *Hematologic Malignancies* and then Ian, Julian, and I edited a book on breast cancer. Cancer of the breast is so complicated and so sensitive that we could not limit the authorship to the scientists of a few select institutions. We had to take advantage of the combined knowledge of very experienced investigators and clinicians. My task as first editor was especially daunting because I, an immigrant with English as a second language, had to correct the contributions from French, German, and Italian authors without stepping on too many toes. The chapter written by Dr. Pierquin, a French radiotherapist, was so bad that I returned it to him for a complete rewrite. His second try was equally bad, and I ended up rewriting the entire chapter.

For one meeting in Geneva, Ian, Julian, and I invited our wives to join us, and it was during dinner that Julian showed the symptoms of his own cancer. He had lost weight, required pain medication, and had little energy. He died shortly before the book *Breast Cancer* was published. "He was a man of supreme international repute, a dedicated doctor beloved by his patients, who came from all over the world to seek his advice and care. The study and management of breast cancer was a major part of his working life." Thus wrote Ian in the preface of our book. I remember Julian's disorderly office in the basement of The Royal Marsden and how he was always late, too busy to watch the clock. Ian and I miss a warm friend. Not long thereafter I was elected a Fellow of The Royal Society of Medicine.

The East German government was unable to pay its dues to the UICC and instead invited us to hold one of our meetings in East Berlin. I took a taxi (it was a Mercedes) from Templeton airport in West Berlin, and the driver dropped me off at Checkpoint Charlie on a rainy afternoon. My driver pointed me in the right direction, and I walked, pulling my luggage behind me. An East German guard on a tower followed me in with his binoculars. A soaking wet Dr. Roberto Estevez waited in the rain outside a low wooden building when I arrived.

"How long have you been waiting, Roberto?"

"Two and a half hours."

The border guards processed busloads of teenagers without delay; cars did not have to wait either, and they ignored us. All guards were Germans, and I had not been under the German boot for four years during the occupation of Holland for nothing. I knew their mentality and knocked on the door, a commanding type of knock. A guard appeared, looked me up and down, and snarled a single word, "Warten." In German I told him in no uncertain terms that Herr Professor Estevez and I, Professor Hoogstraten, were the invited guests of the East German government.

"You let us go through immediately or we will leave and inform your government that you had left us waiting."

The snarl changed in tone, and with a "*Jawohl Herr Professor*" we were processed in record time through passport control and customs. Professor Heise, of the cancer institute, welcomed us at the other side. He too was soaking wet. He drove his noisy little car through empty streets lined with dreary gray houses and office buildings. We passed a familiar-looking tram and the sound of its bell reminded me of the streetcars of Amsterdam; the Germans stole enough of them and shipped them to the Reich during World War II. A policewoman on a platform directed traffic around a square. She stopped us, let the only car from the right go through, and waved us on.

The rectangular International Hotel had hundreds of square windows on its four flat sides and no steps leading to the entrance. Dr. Heise showed his identity papers to the guard at the door, escorted us to the registration desk, and asked us to meet him at seven o'clock at the desk. My room was sparsely furnished, there were stains on the carpet and bedspread, and the phone was in the hall near the elevator, attended to by a heavyset woman in a blue uniform. After I took a bath and pulled the plug, the water ran out in record time with loud noises. No wonder—the short outlet pipe drained the water into a four inch round hole in the floor.

Our hosts treated us to dinner in a restaurant atop a high tower from which we had a great view of the city. We could not see the infamous wall dividing West and East Berlin, but it was obvious where it was by the numerous lights on one side and the near darkness on our side. Professor Tannenberger, the director of the institute, welcomed us and introduced the heads of his departments. They were all young, and the director himself was barely forty years of age. I wondered whether the Communist Party had replaced the senior Nazi staff members with inexperienced juniors? We toasted with East German whisky and Russian wine. Tannenberger apologized that there was only one selection for dinner. "There was a large crowd for lunch and the kitchen has run out of supplies."

The tower stood near a square at the crossing of six wide streets.

"I hardly see any cars on the roads," I remarked to my neighbor.

"Today is a big holiday," Tannenberg quickly replied for him, too quickly. "The people like to eat at home during holidays."

The next morning on our way to the cancer institute we again saw very few cars. "It must be another holiday," Julian said dryly.

The Zentrale Krebsforschungs Institut, renamed the Robert Roessle Hospital and Tumor Institute after the wall came down, stands on Lindenberger Weg 80 in a pleasant wooded area on the northeast outskirts of Berlin. Robert Roessle had been a famous pathologist in Berlin. He founded the institution that now bears his name in 1956. Tannenberger welcomed us on the top floor, which housed a permanent exhibit of the eight research projects conducted in the institute. "Can I answer any questions before we start?" he asked.

"Is this the only cancer institute in Berlin?" Julian wanted to know.

"It is the only cancer institute in the country."

"Then you must be very busy," I said. "May I ask how many patients are admitted in a year?"

"I do not know the exact figure, but our beds are always full. We have long waiting lists."

When there were no more questions, he said, "Will you now each select one project and the scientist conducting the project will explain it. Shall we say for two hours?" He smiled and nodded to us one after the other.

"I think that we should rotate. We can easily look at all projects in two hours," I interjected.

My suggestion slightly annoyed him. "Do as you please."

The research projects were terrible, decades behind the time, and the investigators had only shallow knowledge of their subject. One project interested us, and we gathered around the scientist, Professor Heise, who was about fifteen years older than his colleagues were. He knew what he was talking about, and we had a lively discussion to the increasing annoyance of Tannenberger.

"The other projects are also interesting," he pleaded, but we paid him no attention.

At the end of the two hours, Tannenberg took us downstairs to our bus.

"I'd like the see the hospital, if you do not mind," Ian Burn said.

"But your meeting. You will have no time."

Ismail took the director's arm and smiled, "I'll make some time."

We entered the long rectangular hospital through a side door and took the stairs to the second floor. Tannenberger opened the door, and we stared at a long corridor with rows of closed doors on both sides. "There is not much to see," he shrugged his shoulders.

"Could we see a room please?" one of us asked.

"I'll ask the head nurse," but it took him a while to find the door to the nursing station. He knocked, the door opened a few inches, a few words were exchanged, and he was permitted to enter. The door closed, and we were left standing in the corridor.

"Nice inviting place isn't it?" Ian said.

The door opened five minutes later. A starchy nurse gave us an imperious nod and walked to another door. The director made up the rear. There were six beds in a square room with a minimum of furniture. Five beds were immaculately made up, and a patient occupied the sixth; so much for the waiting list. "We had a holiday, the patients went home," Tannenberger tried, but we had heard enough lies and returned to our hotel for our closed meeting. Ian, Julian, and I decided to ask Dr. Heise to write a chapter on the methodology for hormone receptor determinations for our book on breast cancer. That evening we dined in a large house with elegant furniture and fine paintings on the walls. The house—we were not told who lived in it—was in sharp contrast with the stark surroundings we had seen earlier. Cars were available to drive us back to the hotel, but four of us chose to walk. One department head acted as a guide, which was not a bad idea, because it was quite dark outside.

"Where do you live?" I asked when we were close to the hotel.

"Right there." He pointed to a large building with lights in only two windows. "That light, on the right, that is my apartment."

He did not bring us to the doors of the hotel. Instead he said good night at the corner, and that was a mistake, because the doors were locked. An armed guard sitting on a chair inside waved us off, but when we persisted he opened one door slightly.

"Passports," he demanded.

The others looked at me, but I conveniently pretended not to speak German. Instead I pointed to the registration desk and said, "Our passports are at the desk."

"*Ich verstehe Sie nicht,*" he shrugged and proceeded to close the door. I pushed the door wide open, walked by him and waved the others on. "Let's go." For a moment, they hesitated, but when the surprised guard did not stop them, they followed.

"That was pretty gutsy," said Ian.

Julian looked back at the guard. "He just closed the door and sat down again."

"The guy just tried to be important," I said. "You can do that to a German. I wouldn't have done it with a Russian."

When we looked for the apartment of our guide the next morning, the building turned out to be a factory. It did not take long to pass Checkpoint Charlie in the western direction. I recently called my friend Dr. Peter Hohenberger, a surgeon working at the cancer institute, who told me that Tannenberger had left Germany shortly after the Wall came down.

18

THE ONCOLOGY DIVISION

I was no longer a full-time clinician after 1976. The chairmanship of SWOG and the extracurricular activities, as well as the administration of an ever-enlarging oncology division did not leave me enough time to have a private practice. I had to make a choice between being a regular bedside physician or a part-time clinician with other responsibilities on his plate. I chose the latter. We lived at a time when clinical cancer research was just stepping out of its baby shoes, when surgery, radiotherapy, pathology, medical oncology, and other specialties such as gynecology, urology, and orthopedics began working together, and when we made the first steps toward integrating basic science and clinical research. It was an exciting time of head knocking, pushing and shoving while finding commonalities, learning to respect each other, and making new friends.

Ron Stephens assumed more and more of my clinical responsibilities. He turned out to be an excellent and enthusiastic teacher and a superb physician. He was built like Wasserman: short, strong, a tendency to be overweight, but unlike Lou he was easy to get along with and most of the time in a good mood. However, it was better to stay out of his way when he was angry, because he would let us have it when he thought he was right about something. It was easy to recognize Ron; he was the guy with his coffee mug in hand, the one who admits to at least twenty-five refills a day. He concentrated on tumors of the kidney, bladder, and prostate. He chaired several studies of those tumors, the NCI asked him to go on site visits, and he eventually became the chairman of a study section of the NIH.

I selected the study of new drugs as the major research project for the division. Actually words like *compound* or *agent* were more appropriate, because they had never been used in humans. These so-called new drugs came straight from mice, rabbits, monkeys, and dogs. They had shown some antitumor activity in the animal tumor screen and now it was time to determine what types and severity of toxicity they caused in humans and what dosage was tolerated without too much toxicity. This research was the so-called Phase I study, and about eight institutions in the country were qualified to perform these studies under a contractual arrangement with the NCI.

The University of Kansas was exceptionally well equipped to investigate new agents. Professor Daniel Azarnoff was director of a superb division of clinical pharmacology and clinical pharmacology-toxicology center in the medical school. On the university campus in Lawrence, Professor Tak Higuchi chaired an outstanding department of pharmaceutical chemistry, one of the few in the country. Together we formed a unique team and learned to appreciate each other's work. The basic scientists made bedside rounds with us and came away with new ideas for drug delivery systems. Azarnoff's people helped us find the doses of the drugs, and we provided them with urine and blood samples. I enjoyed going to the clinic and working alongside my colleagues. Our team completed the Phase I studies of several compounds that were then ready for evaluation of whether they had a beneficial effect against any human cancer.

Margaret

We depended on volunteers to conduct these Phase I studies, patients I regard as the most courageous people doctors will ever meet. Margaret was such a patient. She and her husband of forty-four years were both retired schoolteachers. When they came to see me, they appeared to be a well-balanced couple. She had lung cancer, but that did not temper her good mood and easy laugh. She was a small woman, slightly on the heavy side, and she wore somewhat unconventional dresses with a different shawl on each visit. He was quiet man, his white hair with a sharp separation on the right, wearing a neat suit, a tie, a shirt without a button-down collar, and his black shoes were obviously polished every day. Her left lung had been surgically removed, and she had received post-operative radiation therapy. Margaret was referred to us because the tumor had spread to her right lung.

"Margaret, your cancer is of the type that usually is resistant to chemotherapy."

"Isn't there anything?" she persisted.

"Not really. The conventional drugs have had little success. However, we do have a new drug called methyl-CCNU, and we have seen a few remissions in adenocarcinoma, your kind of tumor."

"Well, how about giving it a try?"

I explained the side effects of the drug and its method of administration, and after four doses Margaret was in a partial remission that lasted six months.

"You're coughing again," I remarked when she and her husband saw me in my office one Friday afternoon.

"Yes, and I have lost weight," she added.

I did not have to tell this intelligent woman that she had relapsed; she knew it before she came in. The chest X-ray showed that the cancer had spread further.

"Well, thank you for trying anyway," she said.

"Yes, thank you," her husband added.

"Don't forget, we'll help you all the way," I said on their way out. She smiled.

There was a note on my desk from one of the fellows when I returned from rounds on Monday. "Margaret was admitted to room 312," it read. That puzzled me, because 312 was in the psychiatric wing. I took the special elevator to the third floor, rang the bell of the steel wired door leading to the psychiatry floor, and an aid let me in.

"What happened with Mrs. W.?" I asked the psychiatry resident.

"She shot herself—twice."

"Then what is she doing here?"

"Surgery didn't want her and sent her up to us," he shrugged. "You know, suicide."

Thou shalt not commit suicide; it is against the law. This ridiculous edict was still on the books in some parts of the country, including the State of Kansas. One had to be crazy to commit suicide, and therefore one belonged in psychiatry. The admission note and X-rays showed that Margaret had one bullet lodged against a rib in her left chest and another in the capsule of her spleen. She was lying on her back when I entered her room. She turned her head away when she saw me.

"Did you have to be such a lousy shot?" I said.

For a moment she did not move. Then, slowly she turned to me, her face puzzled as if she was trying to decide whether to cry or to laugh. She cried. I put an arm around her shoulder and waited for her crying to subside.

"You are the only doctor who doesn't moralize with me," she said.

"You didn't answer my question, Margaret."

She wiped a last tear away, looked at me, and managed a smile. "I never did learn anatomy. And I didn't have time to look it up."

"Tell me what happened."

When they came home on Friday, she sent her husband to the supermarket for some groceries. With him out of the way, she went to their bedroom, took a small caliber gun from the drawer on his side of the bed, and lay down. She aimed the gun at her heart, pulled the trigger, and waited to die. "After five minutes I could still think, and I figured that I had missed, so I sat up and tried again, but this time I aimed at a different angle. I waited until I felt some gurgling and was sure that it was blood coming out of my heart. Now I knew that I was going to die and lay down again. That's when my husband came home and found me."

"Margaret, you missed because your heart has shifted after the surgery and radiation."

She smiled. "I feel like such a fool."

"So you wanted to die. Why?"

"Because there's nothing left for me to live for, and I didn't want to become a nuisance for my husband."

"Dear, your husband will never think of you as a nuisance. He is not that kind of man."

"I know, and I feel terrible about it. I made such a mess of it."

"May I make a suggestion?"

"Yes," she tentatively answered.

"Why don't you make your remaining time useful?"

She looked at me quizzically. "What do you mean?"

"I mean that it is possible that you can help some other patients."

"You really mean that, don't you?" She was serious and interested.

"Yes I mean it. You can help with the study of new agents that have never been tried before in patients with cancer. In other words, you can become a guinea pig. We have a contract with the National Cancer Institute to study the effects of new agents in volunteers. Mind you, I said agents, not drugs. We know what the side effects are in animals, but we have no idea what they are in man or how mild or severe a side effect might be. There is only one way to find out, and that's by trying the agent in patients."

"Do I have to stay in the hospital for that?"

"No, not necessarily."

Margaret volunteered. She lived for another five months, most of the time at home, and she completed a trial of two new agents.

"Thank you for giving me back my life," she said at her last visit, on her way home to die. "You were right, it was useful."

"Thank you," said her husband.

In the book by John Laszlo, *The Cure of Childhood Leukemia*, Tom Frei wrote, "The patients you do remember are the ones who had courage." Margaret had courage.

Alice

One patient had an especially gratifying outcome of her disease. When Alice noticed that her abdomen was ballooning, she saw her family physician, who told her that her abdomen was full of fluid. He recommended immediate surgery. The surgeon, who didn't want a flood in the OR, first drained most of the fluid with a tube. When he opened her up he saw a cancerous left ovary and that the lining of the abdomen was studded with metastases. He removed the diseased ovary and referred her to me to me for further therapy. I entered the examining room with a "Good morning" and put her chart on the desk. Alice was sitting on the examining table with her legs dangling over the side, and she supported herself with both hands as she leaned slightly backwards. She owned a farm in western Kansas, and her closest neighbor lived a good distance away, too far to see the house. She was a widow and had little occasion for conversation. She nodded.

"I'd like to know whether I am a candidate for chemotherapy," she said before I even had a chance to examine her.

"Can you tell me how this got started?" I pointed to her abdomen.

"There isn't much to tell," she said quietly.

"Well, when did you first notice that your abdomen was larger?"

She put her left hand to her face, slid the little finger over her lips, and thought a while. "About three months ago."

"And when did you go to your doctor?" I wanted to have some idea how fast the fluid had accumulated.

"Six weeks ago," she talked through the finger.

"And what did your surgeon tell you?"

"Not much." Getting a history from Alice was like pulling teeth.

"He must have told you something." I needed to learn how much she knew about her condition so that I could get an idea of what to tell her.

"He said that I had cancer of an ovary and that he had removed it...and that I had to see you."

As was so often the case the surgeon had left it to the oncologist to give the bad news.

"Alice, when the doctor opened your abdomen, he saw not only the cancer of the ovary but also some small tumors in other areas. Those little tumors caused all that fluid in your abdomen, and your doctor wants me to try to get rid of them. You understand that?"

"You're telling me that the cancer has spread, aren't you?" she said, and her face showed little emotion.

"Yes, it has, and I'd like to give you a drug that may get rid of it."

"What are the chances that I'll respond?" This stoic woman wanted to have everything up front. She had a farm to think of.

"About one in three patients respond. The drug itself has very few side effects, and you'll be able to function normally most of the time."

"Let's go ahead then."

Fortunately, she had a remarkable response. The fluid accumulated slower and slower, and after eight weeks there was none left.

"Alice, you have done very well."

"Thank you, doctor." She smiled, the first time I had seen any reaction. It doesn't matter how good a patient responds to treatment, the anxiety remains for a long, long time and sometimes never goes away.

"Now we have a little dilemma. How long should you take the pills? There are no hard and fast rules to go by—three months, six, a year? I honestly don't know, but at least we are fortunate to have the dilemma."

"I am grateful," she said. "The good Lord is looking after me."

"Why don't we take the middle road and continue the pills for six months?"

"I'm in your hands."

Alice took Melphalan for six months and then dropped out of sight. Two years later she walked into my office without an appointment, but again with a hugely distended abdomen.

"I won't ask you where you have been," I said, "but you have a problem."

"I know."

She sat at the edge of the chair with her legs spread to accommodate her abdomen and fidgeting with her purse. She looked down at her hands and now and then glanced up at me.

"Why don't we forget what happened after your last appointment, shall we?"

"I'm sorry."

"Now how long has this been going on?"

"About a month."

"Can you climb on the table?"

My nurse and I assisted her, and the first thing I noticed when she lay down was that her abdomen didn't sag. The flanks did not bulge and on percussion she sounded hollow everywhere.

"You have an awful lot of gas in your belly, Alice."

"You mean there is no fluid?"

"Not as far as I can tell, just air. We'll take an X-ray."

Thirty minutes later the radiologist called me. "You'd better come and have a look."

I went downstairs.

"I've never seen anything like it," he said.

The film showed massive distention of the bowels, no free air, and no fluid. However, in the left lower side was a round, partially solidified object, the size of an egg.

"What's that?" I asked.

"If I didn't know better, I would say that she has swallowed a stone."

"I may have good news for you Alice," when I came back. "From the X-ray it does not look like the cancer is back."

She closed her eyes, took a deep breath, and let it out. "Are you sure?"

"No, I can't say for sure, but let's hope so. However, your colon is blocked off and you need to have an operation. Soon, before you explode. Tomorrow, I would say, or, if I can arrange it, today."

"I'll do whatever you say."

I called the Dr. Allbritton, the chairman of surgery, and explained the situation.

"I can do her tomorrow," he said. "Why don't you admit her?"

Alice went straight from my office to the admission office and was in surgery the next day. I sure did not envy the surgical team when they opened her abdomen and they had to let all that gas escape. Allbritton called me with the outcome. "She had a fecalith the size of an egg. It must have been there for a quite some time to accumulate that much calcium. Then it finally got stuck. There is no sign of cancer anywhere."

I went to see her in the recovery room. "Alice, all you had was a partially calcified piece of stool that had become stuck. There is no cancer."

"That is good to know," she replied without the least amount of enthusiasm or relief.

She disappeared again after she left the hospital, this time for good.

John

Another patient also disappeared and returned, but it was quite unexpected. I had seen many patients with multiple myeloma at Mount Sinai and had reviewed the charts of all patients with myeloma in the record room. I did the same with the cases at the University of Kansas. Together there were more than five hundred cases, and with that many I would be able to learn whether the survival time had changed in the last fifty years. I could find out whether better patient care and new drugs had made a difference. However, I did not have the accurate information of all patients, one of whom I had seen in Brooklyn.

John was sixty-three years old, and he had multiple myeloma, a fatal form of bone cancer. We treated him with the usual chemotherapy, but he had only a partial response. He relapsed, and then the worst thing happened. During a coughing spell he broke his sternum, the breastbone to which the ribs are attached. He now had a so-called flailing chest, because it just flapped with each breath. It is extremely uncomfortable, and, even though John had far advanced cancer, he still needed to have the two halves sewed together.

I explained the situation to John, his wife, and his son, who was a physical therapist.

"It is risky, John, but I still recommend that we let a surgeon try to stabilize your chest. You can't live like this." I had just said the obvious.

John, who did not have the breath to speak, nodded.

"Dad, I agree with the doctor," said the son. "Maybe they can fix it, Dad, and then Mom and I will help you."

So John had the surgery. He stayed in the hospital for another three weeks, and then his family took him home. To die, I was sure, but before he left he told me something remarkable.

"I died on the operating table, Doctor."

"It's a good thing you didn't, John," I kind of joked.

"No, I am serious. I know I died. I found myself floating above my body and looked down. The doctors and nurses working on me, pumping and squeezing. 'Why are they working so hard,' I wondered. Then I knew—I had left, and they were trying to get me back. They tried so hard that I could no longer disappoint them. 'I must go back,' I said to myself. And so I did."

An unlikely story, I thought.

"Are you sure you didn't dream this, John?"

"No, Doctor. That's what happened, and it was no dream."

"Well, then I believe you." I knew better than to argue with a very sick patient.

"Anything happen during that operation on John?" I asked the surgeon a few days later.

"We lost him for a while. I was sure that he was gone, but then he came back."

The surgeon used the same words with which John had described his experience.

It was now eight years later. I had his date of diagnoses, but not of death, and I called his wife in Brooklyn.

"Mrs. Y., this is Doctor Hoogstraten—"

"Oh, Doctor Hoogstraten," she interrupted me with a happy voice. "So nice that you called. Would you like to talk to John?"

Whoops. I swallowed my breath. I was just about to ask her when John had died, but I was saved by the bell. "Yes please."

Her husband came on the line. "Hi, Doc. How are you?" His voice was strong.

"Forget about me, John; how are you?"

"I'm fine, Doc."

"Tell me about it," I asked. "Are you in bed?"

"No, I'm sitting in my easy chair. There isn't much to tell really. My wife takes good care of me, and our son comes over every day to give me some physical therapy. I can't do much, Doc, but I enjoy reading the newspaper and looking at TV, you know."

We talked a little longer, and when I completed my analysis, I marked John as still living. John was not cured, but I wonder, was this also a miracle?

Marian

Then there was Marian. She came to us with widespread Hodgkin's disease involving both lungs and the liver. Ron started her on combination chemotherapy, and she had a good partial remission that lasted about a year. After relapse she volunteered for Phase I trials of new agents. Marian and her boyfriend were students in the Department of Psychology at the University of Kansas, and Ron and I never before had such an uplifting experience as with those two. They were never down, not even when the end was in sight.

"Would you mind talking to our class at the university?" Marian asked one day.

"No, that'll be fine," we said.

"What would you like to talk about?"

"Since you are both study psychology, how about if we talk about the practice of active euthanasia?" I suggested.

"Great," she said.

Two weeks later Ron and I drove to Lawrence, where the chairman of the department welcomed us into his office. "You have quite an audience," he said. "Practicing Active Euthanasia. What a topic in conservative, Christian Kansas."

The conference hall was packed to the rafters with professors and students, far more than there were in the smallish Department of Psychology. Ron leaned over and whispered, "I don't see the police, do you?"

Marian gave the introduction from her wheelchair. "The gentleman on my right is Dr. Barth Hoogstraten, and next to him is Dr. Ronald Stephens. They are my doctors. I have terminal Hodgkin's disease, and I invited them to talk about a topic of their choice. Please welcome them."

There was some polite applause. The air of expectation was palpable in the hall.

"Doctor Stephens and I are medical oncologists, and we treat cancer patients with chemotherapy. Most people associate that word with toxicity—bad side effects—and we are not here to deny that the majority of our drugs have side effects. Marian knows that all too well. However, we also help patients in other ways by treating the symptoms of cancer, and in the end by helping them with the dying. We practice active euthanasia, and from the size of this audience it is obvious that the title of our talk has created some excitement."

Laughter.

"Just what is euthanasia? It is a Greek word combining *eu,* meaning "well," and *thanatos,* meaning "death"—in other words, an easy death. Now, what do Doctor Stephens and I mean by the word *active?* It does not mean the act or method of causing death, of putting an end to suffering. We mean it to be assisting the patient in approaching death, making the process of death as easy as possible."

Ron gave a beautiful talk, as only he could. Direct, warm, and yet not pulling any punches. Not one person left the hall. They had come to hear something exciting, provocative. They left pensive, but not before they came down and surrounded Marian to thank her, because we had made it clear that it was she who made active euthanasia so easy for us. She too was a patient we will never forget.

Art

Art was a three-letter man at Notre Dame, which was not only a rarity, but even more remarkable because he was such a small man. He was a top NCAA executive. Art had an inoperable malignant insulinoma, an exceedingly rare tumor of the pancreas that produced extraordinarily high levels of insulin. His blood sugar was so low that he required continuous infusions of glucose. I had never seen a patient with this tumor and had no idea how to treat him. I called Stephen Carter at the NCI and learned that they were investigating a new antibiotic with a very long chemical formula, forty-two letters long. They called it Streptozotocin for short, only fourteen letters.

"Art, I have never treated your type of tumor before, but I do know that there is no truly effective drug. The National Cancer Institute is looking for patients with malignant insulinoma to study the effect of a new agent called Streptozotocin. In laboratory animals that drug kills the cells in the pancreas that produce insulin, and the question is whether it does the same in man."

"Are you asking me to volunteer for a study doctor?"

"Yes Art, that's what it comes down to."

Being the fighter he had always been, he told me to go ahead. Unfortunately, he did not respond and went rapidly downhill. On the evening before I was to leave for Europe, I went to see him one more time.

"Do you know that Art organizes the NCAA basketball tournaments?" his father-in-law, a retired surgeon, asked.

"No, I didn't. My children follow the games, but I'm not really a basketball fan."

"Tonight is the final for the national championship," his wife added.

"But then you should see it, Art."

There was no TV set on the metabolism research floor, but I found an empty room with a set on another floor, and we moved Art. His wife and the nurse propped him up so that he could see the screen, and the four of us sat down to follow the game. During halftime the announcers analyzed the first half, and then one of them said, "We like to take this opportunity to send our best wishes to Art, who is in a hospital in Kansas City."

"For our listeners, Art is the NCAA organizer of this championship tournament, and we wish him a rapid recovery," said the other.

Art died privately during the second half while we were still watching the game.

"He is gone," his wife said quietly.

"That little trooper enjoyed his last game. Beautiful." The old surgeon's jaw set firmly as he put an arm around his daughter. It was beautiful, because Art had an ever so slight smile on his face, as if he felt their love.

Marian had not mentioned God during her illness, and neither was God spoken of while Art was dying. In thinking about it, I realize that God was not often brought up at the deathbed. Death is a lonely happening; it is personal. Left behind is community faith, as are the priest, minister, or rabbi, who often cannot be present. They become active after the death to comfort those left behind. Recently the members of our small island community went to the memorial service for one of our members, "to pay tribute," they said. Where were so many of them when they could have lent a hand? And why did the substitute priest find it necessary to start the service by saying, "I didn't know the deceased"? Why did he not use her name?

"Wasn't that a nice service?" some people commented later. No, it was not. It seemed so impersonal for someone who had just died. Geert Mak, a Dutch writer whose father was a minister of the Dutch Reformed Church, wrote in his book *The Century of My Father* of how his father had sat up in his deathbed and said, "Am I not dead yet?"

"No, but you don't have long to go," his wife replied.

"Good."

When it was his mother's turn to leave a few years later, she got up from bed, sat between her two daughters at the window, took their hands, and said, "I must look at the clouds once more." She died the next morning. Neither of these two orthodox Christians mentioned God during their last moments of life.

"You do believe in God, don't you doctor?" I have been asked that question several times by patients and family members, and I never gave the straight answer "No, I don't," because that would be have been inappropriate for the moment. Nienke and I put our faith in that what is most valuable in humanity—our actions, not our words or professed faith. In our life, we have no need for God to hold our hands. We place our trust in the beauty of life and accept death as a natural end. My answer to the question has been that I was there to help, which satisfied the questioners.

19

FRAUDULENCE IN SCIENCE

Kings, presidents and CEOs have committed fraud, and so have some doctors and scientists. If properly handled, few people outside the university walls learn about it. My friend Dr. Stephen Schwartz of the University of Chicago was the victim of fraud many years ago. At a meeting of the American Association for Cancer Research, he announced that he had made a cell-free extract from the brains of mice with leukemia. After he injected the extract into the spinal fluid of healthy mice, they too developed leukemia. In other words, he had discovered a yet unknown factor that transmitted leukemia. It was an astounding new finding.

Slowly, ponderously, Professor Ludwik Gross rose from his front row seat, and a deferential audience waited for the great man to speak. "Doctor Schwartz, vee tried but vee can not repeat your vork," he said and sat down.

The *grosse Ludwik* was *the* virus expert, the discoverer of the Gross leukemia virus.

"We'll be happy to show Professor Gross how it is done when he visits our laboratory," replied Schwartz with a smile.

However, Gross's condemning sentence stung. Steve immediately left for Chicago where, after intense questioning, his chief technician confessed the terrible truth. After many years of one failed experiment after the other, she could no longer stand seeing her boss disappointed, and had faked the results without telling him. Steve retracted his report, apologized to Dr. Gross and was never heard of again. The affair was properly handled, did not hit the news media, and I doubt that many cancer researchers know of the episode.

In SWOG, too, we had a problem. Soon after we initiated a new study of acute leukemia in adults, I noticed that MD Anderson entered an unusual large number of patients. All patients were supposed to be randomized among three treatment arms, one of which contained immunotherapy with BCG. In Kansas, we had already entered sixteen patients on the study, but instead of at least three or four cases on the immuno arm, only one was. I smelled a rat and began to ask a few questions. A week later, Steve George from the statistical office in Houston sent me a "For your eyes only" envelope. It contained a copy of a confidential memorandum from Dorothy Abernathy to the staff of MD Anderson, and of the statistical office: "All our patients are to be entered on the immunotherapy arm only. This memo is for our eyes only."

I immediately demanded to see the charts of all patients entered on the study by MD Anderson, and discovered that most patients had received the immunotherapy *before the study started, before the study was filed with the FDA.* The institution had received a one million-dollar grant from the American Cancer Society to study BCG immunotherapy in patients with cancer, and MD Anderson now also claimed credit for entering the same patients on the SWOG study for which it received support from a NCI grant. In other words, they were double dipping. Dr. Freireich was the chairman of the study, and I had kept him on as chairman of the Leukemia Committee of SWOG when I became chairman. Without further ado, I fired him from both positions. I called Chuck Coltman, explained what had happened, and asked him to step down as the chairman of the Lymphoma Committee, and take over the Leukemia Committee. He did not hesitate for a second, something for which I was grateful, and would never forget. Steve Jones succeeded Chuck as chairman of the Lymphoma Committee.

Freireich was a prominent scientist, who would be a future president of the American Society of Clinical Oncology. He demanded a hearing during a closed session of our Joint Executive Committee. I informed the committee of my actions but had given no details.

"You have entered patients on the study who had already completed their therapy as if they were new cases," I began the session. "You did so before the study was activated, and you did not submit your patients to randomization. Your actions have introduced bias that destroys the credibility of a SWOG study, and threatens the integrity of SWOG. You have done so with the full knowledge of the director of the Biostatistical Office, and behind the backs of the other institutions. You are no longer fit to be the chairman of that study, and of the Leukemia Committee."

After this introduction, I gave him the floor. He raved and ranted for about ten minutes, and discredited me as a chairman and investigator. He finished by soliciting questions.

"There will be no questions. You are dismissed," I told him instead.

One of his associates and the group statistician, both members of the executive committee, tried to defend him.

"How can you possibly defend something so outrageous?" an indignant Chuck Coltman said. "This smells like outright fraud."

The committee supported my decisions. All this took place three weeks before SWOG was scheduled for an evaluation of the group's performance by a team of about twelve outsiders selected by the NCI. This site visit was to last three days, and we were well prepared. I intended to start by giving an overview of our accomplishments during the past three years, and then the chairmen of each scientific discipline would go into greater detail. The site visitors had a copy of the agenda, and they had immediately noticed the changes in chairmanship. They had discussed it amongst themselves the evening before. Dr. Denman Hammond, the chairman of the site visit team, approached me before the session started.

"What's going on with Freireich and the leukemia committee?"

"Denny, I'm going to ask that you trust me on this. It is an internal matter of the group, and we took care of it. I prefer not to give any details."

He looked at me for a moment. "OK, Barth, I'll handle it."

During the afternoon session I introduced Chuck as the new chairman of the leukemia committee.

"What happened to Dr. Freireich?" site visitor Dr. Clara Bloomfield asked.

"Dr. Hoogstraten has already explained that to me earlier this morning," Hammond said. "Dr. Coltman, you have the floor."

By our immediate action, we kept the fraud out of the limelight and prevented further damage and embarrassment to SWOG and to MD Anderson.

The immunotherapy in the study consisted of Bacillus Calmette-Guerin, or BCG. This is an altered strain of the tuberculosis bacillus used as a vaccine against tuberculosis. It is thought to stimulate the body's immune system. Dr. Jordan Gutterman of MD Anderson was the recipient of a million-dollar grant from the American Cancer Society grant, and he soon reported the beneficial effect of BCG for patients with melanoma. A year later, at the ASCO meetings, he gave several presentations in which he claimed that BCG also gave good results in patients with cancer of the pancreas, of the stomach, and in four or five other types of cancer.

The name MD Anderson exerts an enormous influence on physicians around the world, especially those in South America. They began giving BCG to all their cancer patients. During a lecture tour in Brazil and Argentina that was all they wanted to hear from me.

"It is only humbug," was my response to their questions.

"Humbug? What is that?"

"It is all nonsense."

"But Dr. Gutterman of the MD Anderson Hospital says that it works."

"I know; I heard him too, and after one of his presentations I told him that it was sheer nonsense."

That is what it proved to be; nonsense. Two years later Dr. John Costanzi presented the results of a randomized study conducted by SWOG in melanoma in which BCG had zero effect. Gutterman claimed that we had used the wrong BCG, but in that too he was absurd. There were over two hundred abstracts of studies with BCG at the next ASCO meeting, the year thereafter barely twenty, and then it petered out to none. BCG was the big lie of the 1970s for us. However, it is not entirely useless, because lately it has been used to treat superficial cancer of the bladder with good results.

Universities and large institutions are ill equipped-to handle fraud within their walls. Presidents and deans tend to move slowly in our litigious society. They are afraid to step on toes and are overly protective of the perpetrators of fraud. The stories inevitably leak out, and when the news media get hold of them the results tend to be disastrous.

In the early 1980s Harvard University was the victim of Dr. John R. Darsee, a young investigator in the cardiac research laboratory. He committed a fraudulent experiment in front of several astonished colleagues and endangered a national study supported by the NIH. His boss considered the fraud to be "a single, bizarre act" and continued to pay Darsee's salary. The dean of the medical school first appointed an in-house investigating committee that whitewashed the affair. The NIH then demanded a thorough investigation by outsiders, and the dean asked some of his colleagues from other universities to form a committee. In line with the old "You scratch my back, and I'll scratch yours" shenanigan that committee's report was wishy-washy. The unsavory affair leaked out and was widely reported in the JAMA Medical News. A furious NIH director, Dr. James B. Wyngaarden, punished the laboratory and criticized Harvard for the way it had handled the affair.

When Dr. Robert Good became the new director of the Memorial Sloan-Kettering Cancer Center (MSKCC) in 1973, he took young Dr. William Summerlin with him from Minnesota. He appointed him chief of transplantation immunology, acting chief of the Department of Cutaneous Biology and Medicine, and made him a full member of the institute. Summerlin reported the successful transplantation of skin from black mice to white mice, but nobody could repeat his experiments. When other MSKCC scientists brought this to Dr. Good's attention, he called for a demonstration, and Summerlin showed him the white mice with black patches of skin. Good looked at them, but he did not touch the mice. Had he done so he would have gotten black paint on his fingers. Again, he and the top hierarchy of MSKCC took a long time to act decisively, and the press took over to the detriment of that proud institution. Good, who had put his protégé in a position that was way over his head, resigned soon thereafter and hasn't been heard of since.

The worst example of fraud was committed in, of all places, the NCI. Dr. Robert Gallo and his associates stole the newly discovered AIDS virus from investigators in the Pasteur Institut in Paris. This story became the subject of John Crewdson's book *Science Fiction* and resulted in a movie about the affair. On April 23, 1984, HHS Secretary Margaret Heckler held an international press conference. "Credit must go to our eminent Dr. Gallo, who directed the research that produced this discovery." The French sued, lawyers of HHS and the NIH denied the theft charges, and the United States Patent Office quickly gave a patent for Gallo's new test for HIV, while at the same time upholding the French application that had been submitted earlier.

Heckler ordered the FDA to award a license for the mass-production of Gallo's HIV testing kit to Abbott Laboratories, and the NIH began paying Gallo an annual fee of one hundred thousand dollars. The test turned out to be a disaster, causing numerous false positive and false negative results. In the meantime the French test proved to be far superior, but according to Crewdson, the Pentagon brass refused to use it because, "It would be un-American for the United States military to buy a French AIDS test." The health of the American soldier was less important than misplaced patriotism.

The people from Pasteur did not give up; especially not after the medical editor of the prominent newspaper *Le Monde* discovered that Gallo had also fraudulently altered a letter from a French colleague. All the while, the directors of the NIH and the NCI failed to act against Gallo and his staff. Instead, they continued to protect him and heaped honors upon him. When several investigations of Gallo's laboratory finally revealed that he had indeed used the French virus, the HHS lawyers caved in and began damage control. After raking in millions annually in patent income, they agreed to give Pasteur half the money. On March 31, 1987, President Reagan and Prime Minister Chirac briskly walked into the Rose Garden of the White House and announced that both countries would share the profits from the blood test. A few weeks later American scientist Gerald Myers of the Los Alamos National Laboratory discovered that all AIDS work at the NCI had been fallacious. The roof fell in at HHS and the NIH, the French won on all fronts, and Dr. Robert Gallo resigned. NIH Director Wyngaarden, who had punished Harvard so harshly, failed to clear up the mess in his own backyard, and his successor, Dr. Bernadine Healy, protected poor Bob for far too long.

The So-Called Breast Cancer Fraud

In the March 13, 1994, *Chicago Tribune* there was an article entitled "Fraud in breast cancer study: Doctor gave phony data over twelve years."

From the March 16, 1994, *New York Times*: "Flawed breast cancer study 'devastates' women."

From the March 28, 1994, *Newsweek*: "How safe is lumpectomy? Flawed breast cancer data raises fear."

On CBS News, Dan Rather—with a serious face, firmed up mouth, and squinted left eye—profoundly announced that officials at the National Cancer Institute had uncovered evidence of major fraud in the most important study affecting women with breast cancer.

Was it true or were these headlines examples of some of shoddy and irresponsible journalism?

No diagnosis of cancer evokes as much emotion, anger, sympathy, and interest as does breast cancer. Women used to have no choice when it came to treatment; they had to have a radical mastectomy. This meant the removal of the entire breast, the underlying muscles, and the lymph nodes in the maxilla, or armpit. The operation left an ugly scar, the ribs were frequently visible under paper-thin skin, and women with small breasts often required a skin graft. The removal of the lymph nodes interrupted the normal flow of lymph from the arm, which could lead to massive swelling of the arm. In addition to the physical scars, the patient was left with a deep emotional scar. She not only worried about the threat to her life but also about her diminished femininity, attractiveness, and loss of self-esteem. She wondered how her spouse would react. Not every husband could or would give her the necessary love and emotional support. Dr. Jimmy Holland of the Memorial Sloan-Kettering Cancer Center in New York City, who has studied this aspect of breast cancer for many years, advises husband and patient to resume early sexual relations as a most important emotional support for the patient.

For a long time the surgeons were satisfied with the results of the radical mastectomy, and the American Cancer Society maintained that radical mastectomy was the only acceptable treatment of breast cancer. When the ACS speaks, people listen. However, not everybody was happy, and in the 1970s investigators in three major centers—Mr. Hayward of the Guy's Hospital in London, Dr. Umberto Veronesi of the National Cancer Institute in Milan, and Dr. Bernard

Fisher at the University of Pittsburgh—reported good initial results with breast-conserving therapy. They met with fierce opposition.

Dr. Jerry Urban at the MSKCC was dismissive of anything less than radical mastectomy. In his chapter of the 1989 book *Breast Cancer* (edited by Hoogstraten, Burn, and Bloom) he wrote, "The tempting sirens of cosmesis, short follow-up, and trendy beliefs call strongly to a shore of folly." It is poetic language indeed. "When the results of careful studies from expert centers, conducted in well-defined, selected populations, are widely and unselectively applied, this shore of folly becomes vast indeed." Urban and his colleagues kept the famous Sloan-Kettering from moving to the forefront of breast cancer therapy. They left a vacuum, and Bernard Fisher stepped forward to fill it.

Bernie and I were fellow cooperative group chairmen, and we have maintained contact over the years. He told me that in 1958 he received a telephone call from Dr. Isidore Ravdin, a towering figure in the cancer world at the time. Ravdin ordered Fisher to go to a meeting at the NCI to participate in a discussion of a trial of chemotherapy in breast cancer.

"Barth, I had no interest in cancer. My research was concentrated in the recovery of the liver after severe injury. But when a man of Ravdin's stature tells you to go somewhere, you don't ask questions, you go."

The participants decided to form a rather loose group of a few interested hospitals, and in 1967 Fisher was elected chairman of what became known as the National Surgical Adjuvant Breast Project or NSABP. Fisher continued, "One day at a meeting of the Breast Cancer Task Force this little guy wearing a raincoat walked in. He took his coat off, which made him even smaller, introduced himself as Nat Berlin, and said, 'Gentlemen, let's do something instead of talking.' I wanted to compare radical surgery with simple mastectomy with or without radiation in women with small tumors, and Nat said, 'OK, let's do it.' That cut off all further discussion, and Berlin promised NCI funding to the tune of thirty thousand dollars."

Bernie was concerned when I quoted him about the little guy with the raincoat. "Don't write that, you know that I would never hurt the man." Nat, who now lives in Miami, always stays a few days with Nienke and me on his trips north. He laughed when I read Bernie's definition of him. "He is right; I am a little fellow. What can I do? And I do remember that meeting, because it was my first one as chairman of the Breast Cancer Task Force."

Early in 1971 Bernie called me, "Barth, tell me about L-PAM."

"What do you want to know about it?" I had published the results of two studies on the treatment of multiple myeloma with melphalan, still known as L-PAM by the surgeons.

"Tell me about the side effects."

"Well, other than an effect on the bone marrow, it doesn't have much toxicity."

"All right, what dose do you recommend?" He talked like a typical surgeon, straight to the point.

"Bernie, what do you want to use it for, and how long do you want to give it?"

He gave me the information, and I recommended a dose that could be given safely over a long period of time. It turned out that he had posed the same questions to several other chemotherapists. The NSABP completed several other adjuvant chemotherapy studies for breast cancer after L-PAM, but the most important studies by far were those with Tamoxifen, a so-called antiestrogen. Soon the whole world knew about these NSABP studies, and just about every woman lauded Fisher.

Then the roof fell in on March 9, 1994, when *Chicago Tribune* reporter John Crewdson called the editorial office of the NEJM and asked what the journal was doing about an obscure report in the *Federal Register* of June 21, 1993. In it the HHS Office of Research Integrity (ORI) reported the results of its investigation of the NSABP. Four days later, March 13, the *Tribune* published Crewdson's story under the headline, "Fraud in breast cancer study: Doctor gave phony data over twelve years." He wrote that Dr. Roger Poisson, chief of oncology at Saint Luc's Hospital in Montreal, had entered women on NSABP studies that were not eligible for those studies. He called it fraud, did not investigate the allegation further, and never gave Fisher a chance to explain what had happened. However, he was proud of what he had done. In a May 8, 2002, e-mail to me he wrote, "As you may know, it was my report in the *Chicago Tribune* of the Poisson case that triggered the Fisher affair. I will be interested to see at some point what you have written about this case."

Where Crewdson goes, Congressman John Dingell, chairman of the House Energy and Commerce Subcommittee on Oversight and Investigations, is never far behind. On April 13, 1994, two weeks after Fisher was removed as chairman of the NSABP, he gaveled his subcommittee to order. He immediately accused Dr. Fisher of mismanagement and charged him with soliciting funds from pharmaceutical companies.

"You spent that money on lavish parties and receptions at the semiannual meetings of the NSABP." Dingell leaned over his lectern, pointed a finger at Fisher, and added, "Meetings in such hardship places as the Doral Country Club in Florida, the Fairmont Hotel in San Francisco, and in a Hilton Hotel. Did you not?"

Fisher tried to say something, but Dingell did not give him a chance. "It appears to me that you are more expansive with your expenditures for parties than you are for auditing."

Bernie was devastated. The charge about the pharmaceutical companies was totally unjustified. I was a cooperative group chairperson for nine years and know that the chairmen did not solicit pharmaceutical companies for contributions. It was the other way around; the companies offered to pay for a reception at group meetings without strings attached. Our members worked hard designing, conducting, analyzing, and publishing the many studies, and they did not benefit monetarily from their participation in the group studies to my knowledge. They deserved an evening of relaxation and intermingling now and then.

NCI director Dr. Sam Broder told Dingell's subcommittee that Dr. Fisher had failed to conduct a timely audit, and, according to an Associated Press report, he said, "Dr. Fisher's response to us was quite disrespectful." Paraphrasing Fisher, he added, "He said 'Who are you to criticize me? I know how to do clinical trials. I've been doing them since before you were a doctor.'" Broder put pressure on the University of Pittsburgh, and on March 28, 1994, Dr. Fisher was fired as chairman of the NSABP after twenty-seven years of impeccable leadership.

Dr. Broder's shabby treatment of Fisher was totally unexpected. "Barth, the university caved in instead of first insisting on a full investigation," Fisher wrote in a May 9, 2002, letter. "Dr. Broder had cordial relations with me as recent as March 7, 1994. He sought my advice on a regular basis about his wife's breast cancer. It was not that I rubbed him the wrong way. Dingell asked questions of the NCI, and they either could not or would not answer them. Consequently, the NCI's oversight was questioned. I was Broder's scapegoat to get Dingell off his back."

Fisher's work affected women worldwide, something Broder failed to recognize. He had succeeded Dr. Vincent DeVita, the man who had supported Fisher for many years and who would have handled the situation decisively. However, Broder was no DeVita. He did not consider the consequences of dragging a flagship NCI project like the NSABP through the mud. His failure ultimately caused great harm to the many women who had put their faith in the NSABP studies.

Nevertheless, he was the director of the NCI, and he wanted to be treated with respect.

In a March 25, 1994, letter to the editor of the *New England Journal of Medicine*, Sam Broder wrote the following.

> The fact that Dr. Fisher and his co-workers published a reanalysis of their results does not relieve them of the simple obligation never to include data from the site of the misconduct and to exclude such data without an explicit disclosure of the nature of the exclusions to the editors and readers of scientific journals. Dr. Fisher also has the duty to notify researchers who may have received specimens of tissues from the site where the fraudulent data was produced.

Broder failed to mention that in 1991 the NSABP had already begun an extensive investigation the matter and that the NCI had explicitly forbidden Fisher from communicating with anybody, including editors and other researchers of the NSABP.

A second letter in the same journal is from Drs. Lyle Bivens and Dorothy Macfarlane of the Office of Research Integrity (ORI).

> Sir, we wish to explain why the ORI did not inform the editors of the *New England Journal of Medicine* why the ORI did not insist that Dr. Fisher publish a reanalysis of the study data immediately. The NSABP chairman and his staff cooperated fully with the ORI investigation once the contact had been made and facilitated the review of all the records.

But was it true?

The answer to that question is in a March 25, 1994, letter to the editor of the *New England Journal of Medicine* submitted by Fisher and his statistician, Dr. Carol Redmond. For reasons only the editors of the journal can explain, they did not publish this letter until May 19, 1994, nor did they apologize.

> It all began in June 1990, when an alert data manager in the NSABP headquarters noticed two different dates in two identical operative reports of a patient who was entered in the study by Dr. Poisson on protocol B-18. [This was four years before Crewdson's article appeared] Three members of the NSABP headquarters staff then went to Montreal and examined the records of all 354 patients enrolled by Poisson in protocol B-06, as well as a random sample of records of patients participating in eight other NSABP studies. They found five records in which the dates were altered. These patients would

have been ineligible for the study at the time of randomization. On February 6, 1991, Fisher suspended Dr. Poisson from entering new patients and immediately notified the project officer at the NCI of the problem. On February 12, he asked Dr. Dorothy Macfarlane, the chief of quality assurance and compliance at the NCI, for assistance in determining what course of action he should take. The ORI instructed Fisher and his staff not to discuss the matter, not even with his own executive committee. It was a full embargo.

The NCI did not uncover the "major fraud," as Rather said on CBS; it was Fisher who told the NCI about it, and it was he who asked for assistance.

Two years later the ORI sent its report to the University of Pittsburgh Office of Research Integrity, but did not send a copy to Fisher. On April 26, 1993, the ORI finally notified Fisher that it had lifted the embargo. A summary of the report appeared in the *Federal Register* of June 21, 1993, and it was that summary that caught the eye of John Crewdson. If he had taken the trouble to ask Fisher what was happening, Bernie could have filled him in about the truth of the matter.

Fisher sued the NIH, the NCI, the ORI, the Department of Health and Human Services, and the University of Pittsburgh, and it did not take long for United States District Court Judge Ricardo Urbina to rule in Fisher's favor. The chancellor of the University of Pittsburgh, Dr. Mark A. Nordenberg, said in a *New York Times* interview that "the dismissals of the misconduct charges resolves one of the final chapters in the case" and that "he was pleased." The university paid Fisher $2.45 million and NIH paid $300,000. Moreover, just as they do in big business, the NIH and the university added a rider that "the settlement does not constitute an admission of liability or a violation of any law, rule or regulation."

Fisher did not exactly become rich from the settlement. "Let me tell you, Barth, most of it went to the lawyers who represented me over the years, and much of the remainder was paid to the US Government as income tax."

The university issued a press release stating that it "wished to apologize to Dr. Fisher and wished him success as he continues in his position of Distinguished Service Professor and Scientific Director of the NSABP." The NIH merely stated that it would consider Dr. Fisher for top advisory committee positions, "taking into account his achievements and reputation." Sam Broder resigned as director of the NCI and now works for the Celera Genomics Corporation. Instead of lending support to the thousands of women with breast cancer, NIH Director Bernadine Healy, who had already flunked with Gallo and AIDS, remained mum throughout the affair. Dr. Bernard Fisher closed the so-called fraud with these words: "The great tragedy is that women in this country thought that the work I did all these years was not credible. They questioned their therapeutic decisions and suffered anxiety needlessly."

And that, John Crewdson, is what I have written about the case.

20

LIVING IN EGYPT AND KUWAIT

In 1978, after seven years on the job, I had earned a rest in the form of a sabbatical, which I could take anywhere in the world. Nienke and I talked it over, and we decided to go to Egypt, where she would meet a culture entirely new to her. My friends Drs. Ismail Elsebai and Nazli Gad El Mawla were excited when they learned that we had chosen their country and their institute. Nazli found a house for us in El Ma'adi, the fashionable suburb south of Cairo where most foreigners lived, but we wanted to be in the city and experience the Egyptian people close up. Nazli then secured what she called a beautiful apartment in Garden City, close to the heart of Cairo. "The president of the University is your neighbor," she wrote. "It will be clean and ready for you when you arrive."

The University of Kansas paid my salary for six months, but I wanted to go for a full year and received a senior international fellowship from the Fogarty International Center of the NIH for the other six months. Frank already had his own apartment in Topeka, Kansas, and Evelien stayed home to continue her study at the music conservatory.

I went first to prepare for the arrival of Nienke, Marion, and Nick, and it was a good thing I did, because Nazli's definition of clean turned out to be filth beyond description. Little children had left hand imprints of their feces on the walls and dirt was piled up in every room. Worst of all there was no air-conditioning. Then there was the kitchen, with tar on the ceiling and thick, sticky brown oil on pans, sink, furnace, and utensils. However, first I had to find out from whence the thousands of cockroaches were coming. The back door of this third floor apartment opened to a three-foot square platform loaded with garbage left by our neighbors, four Koreans who served their army time as construction laborers on the large buildings that mushroomed all over the city. The garbage stank of rotten fish and was covered with nervous cockroaches. With three cans of Raid I built an inch-high wall along the doorstep and used two more cans to kill the beasts around the apartment. Cleaning the rooms and kitchen took several days, lots of soap, buckets of water, bed sheets to serve as rags, and it wrinkled the skin of my fingers. An all-purpose store provided new sheets, pillowcases, and towels. The few pieces of furniture got a firm scrubbing, and after I washed the windows the place was ready for my family to arrive.

The apartment had no telephone, and, even if it had, it would not work because looters constantly dug up the lines and sold the copper on the black market. My contact with Kansas was by telegram, and Nienke was supposed to send one with the date that Marion and Nick would arrive. I arranged to meet them, relaxed after that hard work on the balcony with my feet up and a beer in hand, and enjoyed the view of the garden across the street.

The door opened, and there were a teary-eyed Marion and a somber Nick.

"Thanks for meeting us at the airport, Dad," Marion said.

Somehow, they had managed to direct a taxi driver toward the Meridian Hotel, and the man at the newsstand had told the driver about where he thought I lived. Doormen along the way pointed to our little street, and the last one excitedly told them that this was where the tall doctor lived. That night the doorbell rang, and a messenger from the telegraph office delivered Nienke's telegram twenty-four hours late. He held out his hand for baksheesh. The next morning we bought three flyswatters and had a competition with prizes for the first two places. Marion won with the most flies killed, and Nick managed to hit four with one swat. I treated them to dinner and ice cream at the Meridian. Nick signed up for an Arabic-English speaking high school on El Zamalik Island, and Marion enrolled at the American University.

Nienke came four days later, and she quickly put the apartment in working order as only a woman can. Qasr El Aini—the major shopping street of Cairo—was one block over, and she bargained for everything, just as she had learned to do in Indonesia. She spoke English, the shopkeepers spoke Arabic, both used their hands, and it was a toss-up who enjoyed it more between her and the shopkeepers. The meat hung out in the open air at the butcher shop, and she shuddered when he nonchalantly shooed the numerous flies away with his hand. They made a deal—she indicated the part from which she would buy the meat, and he wrapped it in cloth beforehand. In between, the flies had their way.

The president of the University did not exactly live next door; he lived three blocks down. Our apartment was in Garden City, one of the better neighborhoods. We lived on Shari El Salamlek, a street that was one quarter of a mile in length. The Italian Embassy was on one corner, the apartment building on another, and our balcony looked down on the large garden of the Saudi Arabian Embassy across the street. We were two short blocks from El Corniche, the wide boulevard that runs along the Saiyalet El Roda, a narrow branch of the Nile River that separates Roda Island from old Cairo. The Fontana Bridge to Roda led directly to the Meridian Hotel where we would buy the *Herald Tribune* and have coffee and cake on Sunday mornings. The Cancer Research Institute was within walking distance, five blocks down on the Corniche.

Our building had a doorman, or bawat, and his name was Basha. He was a middle-aged man dressed in a dirty galabia, missing teeth, and with a huge hernia in his right groin that he insisted I should see and feel now and then. There was also an elevator for three people and no more that only Basha was supposed to operate. The bell didn't work, so we yelled, "Bashaaaaa! Bashaaaaa!" when we wanted him to come up. The speed with which he answered depended on his mood and on the size of the baksheesh that he had received that week. The apartment owner lived on the second floor. She was an old woman named Mrs. Hakim who lived with her daughter. Her grandson Cherif and his German shepherd Gypsi lived on the top floor. Basha usually came running when the daughter yelled for him with a short, sharp "Basha." However, on days that she lashed out at him, the elevator mysteriously broke down, and then she too had to walk.

One day Nienke forgot to give him baksheesh and he let her walk up three flights with the groceries. The next morning I took him aside and rattled him with, "Don't you ever let the misses walk up again. If you do I'll talk to President Sadat and have you fired." Basha immediately understood English. I also convinced him that, as a doctor, I had to know where the main switch for the elevator was, and he showed me his secret. After that he never let us wait again.

One day Nienke had a serious complaint. "Do you know what the lazy no good grandson of Mrs. Hakim does?" she said when I came home.

"No, what does he do?"

"He lets that dog poop on the roof. I don't mind walking between dry poop when I hang the laundry, but it rained today."

It rained three times while we were in Cairo, including the day that eight drops fell on my windshield.

"Why don't you talk to Mrs. Hakim?"

Nienke walked down one flight, knocked, and the daughter opened the door.

"Oh, how nice to see you. Come in please."

Old Mrs. Hakim sat bent over in her chair at the table. She gave a toothless smile. The daughter insisted that Nienke have some tea and a biscuit. The table was dirty, and a large cockroach slowly made its way across.

"We have a visitor," Nienke said, whereupon Mrs. Hakim nonchalantly flicked the cockroach off the table with thumb and index finger.

"What can I do for you?"

"It's about Cherif and his dog." Nienke explained her predicament.

"Not to worry." The daughter seemed genuinely annoyed. "I'll talk to him."

However, their darling son refused to get rid of the mess, because that was beneath his dignity. Basha also refused, and after a prolonged fight the daughter ended up doing it.

"Guess what," Nienke said a few days later. "The poopies are gone."

"You have your own toilet," Nazli said proudly when she showed me my office. "And an air conditioner." The office had a desk, a chair, a small bookcase, and the ubiquitous non-working telephone. The toilet had no light. I tried a new bulb, but that didn't work either. So I kept the door ajar, initially to the dismay of Charlie, a huge cockroach. He and I became good friends, and we made a pact: I promised not to disturb him, and he promised to remain discreet. We lived happily together, until the day I closed the door too fast. There was a light crackling sound, and Charley lay crushed between the door and the post. I gave him a proper funeral: a flushing of the toilet.

Cairo had the only cancer research center—that also happened to be the only one in Egypt—and many patients came from far away. They arrived in grossly overloaded buses, in donkey carts, and on self-made platforms pushed or pulled by relatives and friends. They endured enormous discomfort during their journeys and then waited for hours, slowly moving up in the line in the street off the clinic. Once inside the crowded lobby they waited again for a clerk to call their name and then entered the clinic area through that one door. There they waited patiently for a doctor to see them. Never before had I seen such advanced disease. Nazli assigned one of her fellows to work with me who taught me Arabic, and he learned oncology from me. We worked in the oppressive heat from eight in the morning to two in the afternoon, washed our hands at the only sink, and dried them with the only towel. In addition, I felt like a real doctor, not like the one who used to see clean patients in air-conditioned rooms, one at a time. Moreover, I sure welcomed that siesta after lunch.

More than two hundred million people in Africa, Southwest Asia, and the Southern Asiatic countries are infected with a worm called Schistozoma. The word derives from the Greek word *skistos* for split or cleft and *soma* for body. The male worm has a deep cleft in ninety percent of its body, which is from one to two centimeters in length, and with it he embraces the thinner and much longer female. Together they live for up to thirty years in the veins of the human liver and cause a disease called Schistosomiasis, or Bilharzia, after Theodor Bilharz (1825–1862), a German helminthologist, or "one who studies worms."

After copulating, the male carries the female against the blood flow to the veins of the small or large intestine or to the veins of the bladder. There the female deposits between three hundred and three thousand eggs a day, and the eggs begin to destroy the surrounding tissue. They penetrate through the wall of the colon or bladder and are excreted, often in irrigated fields. The egg quickly matures into a larva that finds its way into a snail and begins to reproduce itself asexually into the thousands. About a month later the snail expels the larva into the water, where it penetrates the skin of a farmer working his field, finds a blood vessel, and goes—via the lungs and heart—to the veins of the liver, where it matures to a male or female worm. Dr. Bilharz figured this lifecycle out when he was only twenty-seven years old.

Forty-five percent of all cancers in the Egyptian male are of the bladder, caused by the eggs of *Schistozoma hematobium*. The old Greek word for blood is *haima* and *bio* means life. The word *hematobium* was added because the victim has blood in his or her urine, not because the worm lives in blood. It is said that when Napoleon was in Egypt and saw that so many of his soldiers had red urine, he suspected that it had something to do with the water, and he ordered his soldiers to wear boots when they entered the water.

The chance to study this enormous reservoir of patients with bladder cancer was one of two reasons that I chose Egypt for my sabbatical leave. The other reason was that Egyptian surgeons and radiotherapists insisted that breast cancer was the most frequent cancer seen in Arabic women. In November 1978, I flew to Kuwait to study breast cancer in Bedouin women at the invitation of the minister of health. The country is only ninety-five miles long and forty miles wide. At dinner one night with a colonel of the Kuwaiti air force, I asked him about flying his American-made fighter jet.

He laughed, "There are days that we only take off to the south, to the Persian Gulf, otherwise we're over Iraq, Iran, or Saudi Arabia before we know it."

The population of Kuwait was about one million at that time, of which half were foreign workers and their families, especially Egyptians and Palestinians. For my stay of six weeks, I had a car and a chauffeur with white gloves because the steering wheel was too hot to handle with bare hands. Three things struck me on arrival: First, all houses had a television antenna in the form of the Eiffel Tower that was between ten and twenty feet high, although some were even taller. The Frenchman who sold them on that idea must have made a fortune. The second was a huge building under construction near the end of an enormously wide boulevard. A large sign read, "Kuwait City—Home of the world's largest ice skating rink." Nobody skates in Kuwait, but some American did one hell of a job convincing the Sabah family that the country badly needed a place for the citizens to skate. Third, there were the many green and white container trucks; white for bringing clean water to the houses, and green for collecting the dirty water. Kuwait has no running water and depends entirely on the world's largest desalinization plants.

The original population was Bedouin, who are nomads who move from one oasis to another with their herds of sheep, goats, or camels. They call themselves "people of the tent." Their large, low-slung tents are more than homes; they also serve as meeting places. In that sweltering heat one would expect the tents to be white, but interestingly they are almost black on the outside, because they are "houses of hair" from camels and goats. Bedouins are more concerned about the nights, when the temperature can drop as much as sixty degrees, and it can be quite cold in the desert.

The Bedouins were very hospitable when I visited them to ask them about health issues, but I was careful not to mention the breasts of their women. I sat on rugs in the shade of the open tent and drank tea. I was not permitted to interview their women myself, but the nurse was able to obtain the much-needed details from them, such as how old they were when they had their first menstrual period, how soon they had married thereafter, and when their first child was born. They of course breast fed, but I needed to know how long they had done so. I also wanted to know how old they were at menopause and whether there was any breast cancer in the family. Other questions included how long it had been before they saw a doctor and how long they had to wait before they were treated. The data was quite reliable; however, just like the poorer people in Egypt, few Bedouins knew how old they were. They shrugged their shoulders and just guessed; it's not important in a land where time stands still, where every day is the same.

From the excellent health care statistics in Kuwait, I could establish an accurate incidence rate of breast cancer in these native women and learned that it ranks amongst the lowest reported in the world. That was as I had expected, because Kuwaiti and Egyptian women deliver a full-term first child at a much earlier age than American or European women do and that early age exerts a definite protective effect against the development of breast cancer. Twice as many American women than Arabic women never give birth, Arabic women, and only four percent of women in New York City give birth before the age of twenty, compared to forty-nine percent of Kuwaiti women, of whom many deliver before age fifteen. Our findings amazed the Egyptian physicians and eliminated a myth. The delay in therapy was considerable for Arabic women; only forty-seven percent received treatment within four months after they saw a doctor, compared to eighty-one percent for American women. As a result they presented with much larger tumors.

The day before I was to return to Egypt, I had dinner with Dr. Youssef Omar of the Radiation Therapy Department of Sabah Hospital. He handed me a check for one thousand Kuwaiti dinars.

"What's that for?" I asked, amazed because no money had been mentioned when I agreed to visit Kuwait.

"It is a thank-you from the minister of health."

"But I didn't do much," I protested.

"Yes you did. You made rounds with us, you gave lectures, and you honored Kuwait with your presence." Youssef bowed slightly, extended his hand across the table, and smiled.

"Well thank you, and thank the minister."

Cashing the check was another matter. For that I had to go to an office in the Department of Finance. The waiting room had chairs along the walls, and three men were already waiting. "Welcome to the club," an Australian said.

"I'm just here to cash a check," I said.

"So are we, friend," a Scotsman replied.

"This gentleman has been here three days, he two days, and this is my fourth day," a gentleman of apparently East Asian origin added.

"Does that door lead to the cashier?" I asked no one in particular.

"Yes, and you are to wait here until they call you," the Australian again.

"We'll see about that." I opened the door to a large space with more than thirty desks and a glass-enclosed office in a corner. All heads went up and followed me as I walked to the enclosure. "Are you the paymaster?" I asked the Kuwaiti behind the desk. My Arabic was fairly good by that time.

"You cannot just walk in here. You must wait for your turn," he commanded.

"No sir, I will not wait. This is a check from the minister of health." I put the check on his desk. "Now, do you pay me or do I call the minister?" He paid.

"I'll see you gentlemen," and I waved the money to three astonished men in the waiting room. The Kuwaiti dinar came to 3.25 US dollars in banks, but I traded much better on the black market in Port Said.

After I returned to Cairo, Mrs. Jihan Sadat, the charming wife of the president of Egypt, invited me to tea. In 1949, at age sixteen, Jihan Safwat Ra'ouf became the second wife of an army officer who was fifteen years her senior, captain Anwar al-Sadat. She received me in a large room furnished only with a small gold lacquered table and two chairs. We shook hands, a servant brought a tray, and my hostess poured the tea, which we drank over small talk. We posed for an obligatory photograph to document this auspicious occasion, and then she came down to business.

"I am president of the Egyptian Cancer Society, and I would like to discuss some matters with you. For instance, as you have noticed, Egyptian men are very heavy smokers, and we have a lot of lung cancer in this country. How can our society begin a campaign against smoking?"

"You can begin by cutting down on the advertisements. There is a Marlboro cigarette poster on every tree in Cairo, and that's a disgrace."

"I couldn't agree more with you, and I'll talk to my husband about it." She made a note of it. "What else do you recommend?"

"Egyptian and Kuwaiti women wait far too long before they see a doctor after they find a lump in their breast and unfortunately many doctors do not immediately refer them to a surgeon. The Cancer Society can do a much better job promoting self-examination of the breast, and perhaps you can address the doctors about expediting referrals during your annual meeting."

"May I make a suggestion?" she said. "I'd like to appoint you to our board, and then you can address the board about your concerns at the meeting next week. It is much better that the members hear it from you directly."

President Sadat made a brief appearance before the meeting started. "I hear that you do not like the cigarette posters, doctor." He was smoking his pipe when he said it.

"That's right, Mr. President. The posters promote smoking, and the incidence of lung cancer is already very high in Egypt, sir. Besides, they are unsightly and create a false impression."

"Well, then I better keep Mrs. Sadat happy," he smiled and left. The next morning all posters were gone, removed overnight on orders of a benign dictator.

On the outskirts of Mansura, a city the population of which has exploded to over a million since 1945, time seems to stand still, as it does in most Egyptian towns and villages. The bricks for building the houses come from the many factories that ravage the valuable topsoil left behind after the annual floods of the Nile. The floor inside a typical farmhouse is made of dry mud with a depression in the center for a cooking fire. Along the walls are clay elevations that serve as benches. The donkey and camel are stabled next door, and the roof is stacked high with fodder for the animals and cages for rabbits and doves. Students read their lessons on the street by the light of the moon. There was no electricity or running water and no adequate sewage. I imagine it was similar in the days before Christ.

We went to a newly opened restaurant, were shown a large cage with fat pigeons, and invited to please point to our selection. "No thank you." We politely decided to have lamb instead and sat down for soft drinks and iced tea. Thirty minutes later the smiling waiter refreshed our drinks and brought a salad and bread. After about an hour and a half we began to wonder whether our meal would ever arrive, and then we heard the distant bleating of a sheep. Closer and closer it came, until a smiling farmer appeared on the path next to us. He pulled the front leg of a bleating sheep that hobbled along on three legs on its way to be slaughtered. At least the meat would be fresh.

In that setting, Dr. Ghoneim's accomplishments are most remarkable. He managed to obtain outside funding for a modern kidney dialysis program that is the envy of many European and American hospitals. Ghoneim exemplifies what most leading Egyptian physicians have done. After completing their medical school training they leave Egypt to spend one or more years in places like the Sorbonne in Paris, New York University Hospital in New York, or in reputable institutions in England and Canada.

I asked Elsebai for permission to spend a day in surgery with him.

"Join us tomorrow morning; we have some radical cystectomies."

At seven o'clock in the morning Elsebai, assisted by Mo Mansour and a Canadian nurse, went to work with amazing speed. A radical cystectomy means the removal of the bladder, the lymph nodes, and implantation of the ducts that carry urine from the kidneys to the bladder into the large intestine or through the wall of the abdomen and into a bag. This surgery lasts several hours in the US; the Elsebai team operated on four patients that morning, and only one patient received a blood transfusion during the operation. Elsebai was Sorbonne trained, and Mo had worked in Toronto and at Memorial Sloan-Kettering in New York City.

Aside from our visits to Luxor, Elephant's Island, and Abu Simbal, we had a few special memories and experiences that helped us better understand Egyptian culture. Ancient Egypt was the country of sacred animals, and most sacred of all during the era in which Memphis was ascendant was the Apis bull. Apis, a god of fertility, was also known as the life of Ptah, the creator god of Memphis. The pure black bull was honored for twenty-five years and then slain before it began to show the ravages of old age. It was mummified, mourned for sixty days, and then put in a huge marble sarcophagus. Immediately after the slaying, the priests searched the country for the next Apis bull, identified by secret markings only the priests knew.

The reason for telling this story is because the Egyptians of old had invented the elevator. They buried the heavy sarcophagus fifty feet below ground in the Serapeum at Saqqara, near Memphis. They accomplished this by constructing two identical fifty feet deep pits connected at the bottom by three slots. They filled one pit to the rim with the finest sand, shoved the sarcophagus on top, and with ropes opened the slots below. Under the enormous weight of the coffin the sand flowed through the slots, and while one pit emptied the other filled up. After the sarcophagus arrived at the bottom of the pit, the priests opened a door and used rollers to transport the sarcophagus to its destination. It worked for sixteen hundred years.

A second memorable event was the general election. The trees of Cairo that had been adorned with Marlboro cigarette posters now showed the smiling face of the only candidate, Anwar Sadat. The *Herald Tribune* and American newspapers lauded this "democratic election" as an example for all other Middle East countries.

"Looks like Sadat is going win again," I remarked to Mo.

"Barth, you must understand that politics are different here. Sadat is going to get about 99.5 percent of the votes."

"You must be kidding."

"No, I am not. If it is 99.2 percent, it would mean a bad result."

"When will we know the results?"

"Tonight or early tomorrow morning."

"That's impossible. I can't even call you by phone here in Cairo."

"That's what I mean, Barth. It is all democratic, just like America wants it to be"

"Are you going to vote?"

"Oh sure, and maybe next year sometime they'll find out that I voted."

"So they do check whether you voted?"

"Yes, it may take a long time, but they do keep track."

Anwar Sadat, Nobel Peace laureate and the world's top diplomat that year, was reelected with 99.4 percent of the vote and received congratulations from President Jimmy Carter and other leaders throughout the world.

The third memory is that of the art of giving baksheesh, without which the Middle East could not function. We were walking on the Corniche along the Nile River one Sunday when a policeman on the other side of the six-lane boulevard blew his whistle, stopped all traffic, crossed the street, and held his hand out for baksheesh. We didn't give him any; he smiled, blew his whistle again, and returned to his post on the other side of the Corniche.

Egyptians have made the practice of baksheesh and "You scratch my back, and I'll scratch yours" into fine arts. Honey, Mo's Canadian borne wife, wanted a new refrigerator, and Mo asked me for help. He didn't want to pay the import tax that was approximately equal to the price of the unit. I wrote Cherri Stadalman and asked her to buy a new GE double-door refrigerator with an icemaker and to make sure that it looked like a used one.

"Spill some tomato juice in it or something like that and address it to me." Cherri soon wrote back that the refrigerator was on its way, and we waited.

"Barth, the refrigerator is in Alexandria, but it is brand new," a dejected Mo told me several weeks later. "They want you to pay the import duties on it."

"Even if it is for my personal use?"

"Yes." Mo didn't look too happy. He could have bought the refrigerator for that amount in Cairo.

"I'm sorry Mo, but what can I do about it?"

He threw his hands up. "Let me see what I can do."

"By the way, my international driver's license has expired, and they told me to get an Egyptian license."

"Don't worry, I'll arrange it."

Mo was the principal surgeon of the Egyptian police force, which was a paramilitary unit. A week later he came to my office. "Come with me. We'll get the driver's license." He drove me to the license bureau where a long line was waiting. Mo walked in and came out with an instructor. "He wants you to drive my car."

I got in and backed the car up for maybe twenty yards. Forward, stop, and get out. The instructor filled in the license, and we left.

"Now where do we go?" I had been in Egypt long enough to know that Mo had something up his sleeve.

"We go and see the general. He has to sign it."

The general and Mo were old friends; they shook hands and kissed cheeks. An orderly brought the inevitable tea and Coke, Mo and the general talked, and I waited—for about two hours, while the general worked the phone and discussed some important matters with Mo. Finally the orderly returned, said something to the general, who once more picked up the phone. He smiled, shook my hand, shook Mo's hand, they kissed, and we left without the signature.

"Now what? We didn't need his signature, did we?"

"Now we go to the minister of the interior. Would you mind seeing his wife? She has breast cancer?" He ignored my question.

The minister lived on the second floor on a busy street. Mo greeted him with respect and introduced me. "Doctor Hoogstraten is a famous doctor from America."

Smiling relatives packed the living room. I could not refuse yet another cup of tea, and as usual I waited. The minister left and returned a few minutes later. "Please doctor, follow me."

A very sick woman managed a faint smile. I discreetly examined her. The cancer had spread to the abdomen and skeleton, but before I a chance to talk to her about it, her husband guided me out of the room and into the living room. It was there that he asked whether anything could be done.

"Has your wife received drugs for her disease, chemotherapy?"

She had not.

"You do know that she is very ill?"

They all knew.

"I will try a treatment, but your wife should be in a hospital for that."

The minister readily agreed, as did all family members, in unison, and I said good-bye. On the stairs the minister turned to me and said, "I understand that you have some trouble with a refrigerator. Please not to worry, it will be taken care of."

So that's how the system worked; I owed Mo a favor for the license, the general owed Mo a favor, the minister owed the general a favor, and Honey got her refrigerator without paying import duties. A week later, a messenger brought me a gift from the minister: Gold lettering on blue velvet proclaimed, "Allah Il Allah, Mohammed Rasoul Allah" ("There is no God but Allah and Mohammed is his prophet").

"Guess what?" Nazli was excited when she saw me. "You are going to visit the battlegrounds in the Sinai Desert."

"Wait a minute. What are you talking about?"

"The military has given you permission to go to the Sinai desert." She was serious.

"Nazli, since when do I want to go there?"

"Since I worked it all out."

"You mean *you* want to see the Sinai, and you used *me* to get permission, right?"

"Well, kind of," she said shyly. "But you do want to go, don't you?"

"Sure; can Nienke come too?"

"No, I'm sorry. The officer said no ladies."

"What about you? Are you not a lady?"

Nazli stood up straight and said proudly, "I am a professor."

"Why don't you tell me how this all came about."

Nazli, the only female professor at the cancer institute, was probably the most conservative member of the staff. Her husband was a saintly gynecologist who refused to charge his patients. One daughter studied medicine; the other was, by Egyptian standards, a religious fanatic. Nazli was both provider and housekeeper. As a result, she had seen little of her own country.

"Do you remember you saw my patient with Hodgkin's disease? He is a high-ranking army officer, and I told him that you were interested in seeing the Sinai Desert. He arranged it for Sunday morning. I'll come and pick you up." Nazli was clearly dying to go.

An assortment of about twenty army vehicles lined the curb when we arrived at the barracks. Two weapons carriers led the way, followed by some semi-trucks with refreshments, army trucks with soldiers, jeeps for the officers, and an old staff car for Nazli and me. One vehicle looked like a giant box sitting abnormally high on wheels, and I had no idea what its use was. Off we went down the highway, via Heliopolis to Ismailiya, where it took an hour to ferry our caravan across the southern end of the Suez Canal. We drove south for about forty miles along the Bitter Lakes and stopped where a side road turned to the Mitla Pass. Dark clouds hovered over the mountains in the east.

"Rain, there, rain," our driver excitedly pointed. As aforementioned, it rains two, maybe three times a year in the Sinai.

"How far away do you think those mountains are?" I asked.

He shrugged his shoulders. "Maybe ten miles?"

"I know those mountains," said Nazli. "On the map, they are about thirty miles away."

On October 6, 1973, the Day of Atonement, the holiest day in the Jewish calendar, Sadat unleashed his army against Israel in what is known as the Yom Kippur War, among other names. We were now in the general area of some of the fiercest tank battles. For a while, the Egyptian forces established themselves along the entire east bank of the canal, only to retreat a few days later when Israeli tanks crossed the canal into Egypt and threatened to cut them off. Israel considers this war a qualified failure, having lost 165 tanks and 2,688 men. The tanks are still there, shot to pieces, burned out, gun barrels at grotesque angles, and Stars of David faded by the desert sun. The remnants of Egyptian tanks had long been removed. Nazli could not get enough of walking among the tank skeletons, accompanied by the senior officer and all the while keeping up an enthusiastic conversation. I had seen war before in Europe and the Far East, but in a different setting, with trees, villages, towns, and paved roads. There was nothing here other than sand as far as the eye could see—flat, no trees, only desolation.

Lunch was served; the three officers, Nazli, and I sat in the shade of a truck, and the soldiers huddled in small groups. After lunch the senior officer said something to Nazli.

"He recommends that if you want to relieve yourself, this is the time to do it," she said.

I looked around. "Where?"

"In the truck."

So that is what the giant box on wheels was for, it was our sanitation truck. I then saw that the box had a door in the rear. Two soldiers produced a ladder to gain access.

"Ladies first, Nazli."

She walked to the box, climbed the six steps of the ladder with the help of a soldier, and disappeared. Soon a steady stream of urine clattered from an open pipe under the box and formed a little river in the sand. A relieved Nazli came carefully down the steps.

"Your turn, Barth."

She did not understand why none of the men took their turn in the box, and we were not about to explain the reason why. We relieved ourselves behind a truck.

"Nazli, can you ask the officer where that sanitation truck came from?"

"It's a Russian truck," she reported. That explained the plumbing; I had seen it before, in a hotel in East Berlin.

The commanding officer turned our column around, and we were on our way back. After six miles, we reached a dip in the road at the juncture with another road coming from the east and that's where we came to a halt. The side road had changed into a fast running river, and water swamped our road before continuing on its way to Little Bitter Lake. The top of an army truck rocked in the surging water fifty yards to the left of the road. Its driver and two soldiers had drowned, according to the people in front. Mention the word *desert*, and people visualize a vast landscape with huge sand dunes. However, most of the desert floor is hard as cement and rocky. Rainwater does not sink into it; it runs off for miles toward the lowest point, and that point was Bitter Lake. It had not rained where we were; this torrent came from thirty miles to the east, and all we could do was wait.

An hour later three Swedish UN peacekeepers in a white half-track drove up and looked at the now more slowly moving water. They decided to give it a try.

"How do you know where the road is?" I asked their driver. It was at least two hundred meters through water before the road reappeared on the other side.

"We drive here every day," he said. "It is straight, no curves."

At its deepest point, the water was three feet deep, and they made it without trouble. However, our commanding officer wisely decided to wait another hour because our jeeps would not have made it. When we arrived in Cairo, there was bad news. The rainstorm had passed over the city, and a six month accumulation of fine dust had turned the streets as slippery as if they were covered with grease. The streets of Cairo do not have gutters, and rainwater must find its own way into the Nile River. When an overloaded city bus had hit the slick mud, its brakes could not prevent it from sliding into the Nile, taking its unfortunate passengers with it. Most were feared drowned.

During the sabbatical, I twice returned to the States to chair meetings of SWOG. Flying back from the warm Egyptian climate it was strange to see the snow-covered stretches and the river barges locked in the grips of ice down below. During the second trip, Jim Lowman asked me to accept the directorship of a cancer center that had yet to be created. "The senior executive vice-chancellor wants to discuss it with you."

"That's a new title, isn't it?"

"You might call it a promotion of sorts," Jim said.

"Who is it?"

"Dave Waxman."

"You must be kidding."

Doctor Waxman held the meaningless job of assistant dean for student affairs for many years.

"How did that come about?"

"The new president of the university, Archie Dykes, appointed him."

Dykes had arrived shortly before the start of my sabbatical. He had a Ph.D. in journalism and came from the world of business without any academic achievements. A small man, he quickly began throwing his weight around. He announced that he would maintain an office in the medical school and spend one day a week with us. All he needed was a patsy to follow his orders, and he found one in Waxman.

"We think that you are the right man to establish a comprehensive cancer center," Dave said when Jim and I met him in his small office. "But I want you to understand one thing: This is my desk, and you can not take it away from me." What a strange thing to say.

"What was that about?" I asked Jim on the way out.

"Don't ask me. He is a bit weird, you know."

I should have followed my intuition and refused the job.

21

A TEMPTATION AND A FAILURE

Not much had changed when I returned to Kansas after a year. Ron had firm control over the division, while Cherri Stadalman and Carol Fabian kept the SWOG operations office going. However, they had a surprise in store for me.

"We have a new secretary," Cherri announced the first day after my long absence. "Come in, Andy, and meet the boss."

Andy was now the only male secretary in an office with sixteen women; he was gay, and the girls loved him.

"He is by far the best secretary we have ever had," Cherri said. He was also a graduate of a well-known conservatory and the conductor of an all-male choir.

"Teresa Vietti is on the line for you," a secretary announced.

Teresa was a professor of pediatrics at the Washington University Medical School in St. Louis and the chairman of the pediatric division of SWOG.

"Yes, Teresa, what can I do for you?"

"Barth, the pediatricians of CALGB want to leave that group, and they'd like to know whether there is a place for them in SWOG."

"I'm sure Jim Holland won't like that, Teresa."

"I know, but Jim may be the reason why they want to leave. They think—"

"Teresa, I am not interested what they think. That is between them and Jim. Why don't you invite their principal investigators to our meeting next month, and then we'll talk about it."

"OK, I'll do that. Thanks, Barth."

I buzzed Cherri and our grant and contract manager to come in. "The pediatricians of the CALGB want to know whether they can join SWOG."

"Wow," Cherri. "How many institutions will that be?"

"I'm not sure, but at least fifteen. If I accept them, it'll mean a lot more work for us and for the statisticians. I want you to keep this an absolute secret until I have made up my mind. In the meantime, put on your thinking caps and come up with a preliminary estimate of the additional cost if we include them."

Teresa and I met with eighteen pediatric PIs from CALGB in my hotel suite.

189

"I see several familiar faces, but why don't you start by introducing yourselves, including the name your institution," was how I began the meeting.

"Now, what do you want to know?"

"We'd like to know whether we can join SWOG." They had selected a spokesman.

"Yes, you can. Anything else?"

They were dumbfounded and looked at each other. "Don't you want to know something about us? How many patients each of us can contribute and what kind of research we do besides treating patients?"

"I'll find that out soon enough."

"But some of us have strong programs, and others do not." He still did not get it.

"We have that in SWOG too; haven't we, Teresa?"

Teresa laughed but did not say anything.

"Well, how many of us will you take?" the spokesman asked again.

"All of you."

"You mean—"

"I mean that any of you who want to join SWOG can do so right now, but under one condition—and this is a big 'but': I want you out of here in two years to form your own second pediatric group."

That really surprised them, even Teresa. "When did you come up with that idea Barth, and why?" she asked.

"Well, to begin with, if enough CALGB institutions decide to join SWOG you'll have a big enough body to form a new group. The second reason is that you people do not see solid tumors like lung and breast cancer, and we are moving in that direction more and more in the adult division. The gap between adult and pediatric oncology is widening, and sooner or later, you'll want to be on your own. I'm just giving you a little push."

After waving that carrot in front of our visitors, seventeen PIs decided to join on the spot. The PI of the Mayo Clinic hesitated and later joined the Children's Cancer Group. During the next two years, I helped Teresa set up the Pediatric Oncology Group (POG), recommended that the group take Steve George as its group statistician, and was pleased when he did.

Soon after I became group chairman, I received inquiries from medical schools looking for a new dean. I was also asked whether I was interested in the chairmanship of a department of medicine and even the presidency of a university, but I couldn't work up much enthusiasm for these largely administrative jobs and replied with polite "no, thank you" letters. However, when Donnell Thomas called I listened.

"Barth, the director of our institute is stepping down, and I wondered whether you would be interested."

"I would certainly consider it, Don."

"Good, I'll see what I can do."

About two months later, Dr. William Hutchinson called from Seattle. "Doctor Hoogstraten, we are looking for a new director of the Fred Hutchinson Cancer Research Center (FHCRC), and your name has been brought up. Would you be interested in being a candidate?"

Bill Hutchinson was a wealthy surgeon who established the Pacific Northwest Research Foundation in 1956. His brother Fred was a famous baseball pitcher who later managed the Detroit Tigers, the St. Louis Cardinals, and the Cincinnati Reds. "Hutch" managed the Reds in the1961 World Series, and he worked until he died of lung cancer at age forty-five. A year later, his brother founded the FHCRC in his honor. In 1974, Bill applied for funding to convert the FHRCR into a comprehensive cancer center, and I was a member of the site visit team. He knew how to build the center, and with the assistance of Senator Warren Magnuson had already secured considerable private funding. The new center opened in September 1975 with Bill as the director.

Before accepting the invitation to come to Seattle, I called Don Thomas, who was known for his pioneering work in bone marrow transplantation in patients with acute leukemia and was to become the 1990 Nobel Laureate in Medicine.

"Don, why is Bill Hutchinson looking for a successor?"

"That's a long story Barth, but it comes down to the fact that Bill cannot communicate with us. Can you imagine, in all my years here I have never even been in his office? He also has poor rapport with the directors of the two hospitals nearby, and we depend on them for some of our patients."

"So, will he give up his leadership role?"

"He'll have to; otherwise some of us will start looking for another place to work."

I went to Seattle, talked with the leading scientists, as well as with Bill Hutchinson. He was willing to step down as director and continue as chairman of the board. "I'll just stay in my little office," he said. He showed me two empty floors in a separate building that could house the SWOG Operations Office, and the university could provide the statistical support. I also spent two hours with the director of the Swedish Hospital, one of SWOG's member institutions. He too looked forward to a new FHCRC director to work with. At the end of my visit, Bill asked me to come back for a second visit.

On the plane back I listed the pros and cons of going to Seattle. The pros were many: The physical setup of the center was great; the science was superb; the University of Washington had an excellent reputation, and I had a few friends there; Seattle is a great city; and, most importantly, the scientists were looking forward to the change. There was only one con: Bill Hutchinson was clearly a tough man with whom to deal. With him in his "little office," which I had not seen, I believed he would be looking over my shoulder.

During our second visit, they showed us the sights. Don and his wife had us over for dinner, during which I heard a lot more. A wealthy board member entertained us on his yacht, and a pleasant real estate agent took Nienke on a house tour. I attended the weekly conference of Don's bone marrow transplantation team, and the Swedish Hospital promised beds for my patients.

"That's an impressive mountain," I said to Bill, referring to a painting of Mount Rainier.

"That view alone will cost you ten thousand dollars of your salary," he replied.

"You're wrong. This is my fifth day in Seattle, and I have not seen it yet. It has rained every day, and it'll cost you an extra ten thousand to get me here."

That night Bill took us to his home for dinner. He did all the talking, and Mrs. Hutchinson just sat there. He worked himself up about "those damned liberals" and the "Negroes," and Nienke and I were quite uncomfortable. The next morning I met with the board.

"Doctor, what do you think the center needs most?" one member asked.

"An endowment. The center has little on which to fall back."

"Can you tell us in more detail why we need an endowment?" he persisted.

"The research program is entirely funded by grants and contracts, which is great as long as the country is in the current economic high. However, suppose that the source of funding dries up for one of the programs. The center will then have to sustain it while the director of the program tries to obtain funds from another source. Right now, you do not have the money to do that. In addition, what happens when the center has an opportunity to venture into an exciting new program, and you do not have the space for it? Again, there is no money to build the space." Heads nodded here and there.

"Can you give us some idea of how much you think the endowment should be?"

"I would have to look into that, but offhand I would say at least fifty million."

There were a few more nods, and I left with the impression that the interview had gone well. That afternoon Nienke and I were shown some apartments and houses, and we had a quiet dinner together that evening. The next morning Bill handed me a large envelope. "This contains your contract. Look it over and give me a call Monday." He did not add that he hoped that I would take the job. Don drove us to the airport.

"Did he bring up the liberals and blacks?" he asked.

"Yes. Is he always like that?"

"Whenever he can, but don't let that stop you from taking the job. We really would like to see you as our new director. We need you."

Nienke was quiet on the flight back.

"What are you thinking about?" I asked.

"It rained every day, and the ladies told me that it rains or drizzles from October to April. One of the reasons we left Holland was because it rains so much."

I thought about it over weekend and came to a decision. I would have loved to take the offer, but Nienke's happiness was more important. I returned the contract unsigned, and when I called on Monday morning, Bill's secretary took the message.

The cancer center program at the medical school was in a sad state of affairs when I came back from Egypt. Dr. Loren Humphrey, the chair of surgery, had volunteered to write the grant request for the center, and Waxman gave him the go-ahead. Humphrey liked round figures; he asked for two million dollars, included one hundred ongoing research projects, a list of fifty "scientists," and designated twenty thousand square feet for research laboratories and offices. More than half of the so-called research projects were figments of his imagination, including eight in my name of which I had no knowledge. He listed me as the director, and I had no idea why the NCI bothered to make a site visit.

"Barth, what should we do with this?" the chairman of the team asked before the meeting started.

"Beats me. I only saw it when I returned from my sabbatical."

"Is there any chance for a program?"

"Not when the administration handles it like this. At most I would suggest some administrative support for the director and a recommendation to resubmit a request at a later date."

"That sounds like a reasonable solution. We'll make it a short visit."

That is how the program got off the ground. I asked the personnel office to look for candidates to fill the position of administrator, and—in typical State of

Kansas fashion—they came up with a list of eight retired military men: three brigadier generals, two navy captains, and three full colonels. They all told a similar story about their career in the service, and my comment was the same when they were finished: "I served as an officer in the army, and I know that when there is trouble there is always someone of higher rank on whom to fall back. Was that your experience too?"

The first six candidates replied with almost identical words, "That's all part of the system, but I wasn't like that."

Number seven, a colonel, reacted differently. He stood up and said, "I didn't come here to be insulted. I want you to know that I am proud of my army career, sir! Good day, sir!" He turned around and walked to the door.

"Just a moment please. I'd like you to take the job."

He was just the man I needed, someone who did not hesitate to act on his own and tell me about it later. Waxman promised us office and laboratory space in a building originally assigned to the chemistry department, but even though the space had stood empty for years, the administration refused to release it while the Spanish chairman of the department was on prolonged leave in Spain. I had enough and went to see Waxman.

"I've waited long enough; make up your mind, Dave."

"I can't. My hands are tied as long as he is in Spain."

"And how long is that?"

"I don't know."

"Then call him up."

"What do you mean, call him up? He may be anywhere in that country."

I slammed a fist on his fancy cigarette case. "Damn it, call him right now."

"You smashed my box," he wailed.

"Now, Dave!"

His secretary had no trouble getting the chairman on the line. "Emilio, I have Dr. Hoogstraten in my office, and he wants to know when you can release the space?"

He listened. "I see. I'll go ahead then."

We moved in two days later.

The amount of cancer research in most departments was negligible, and I decided that our best bet for a top-notch program should center on the development and testing of drugs and to forget about a comprehensive program. The main campus of the university is in Lawrence, thirty-eight miles west of Kansas

City. Ron and I already had a fine working relationship with Professor Takeru Higuchi and his staff in the Department of Pharmaceutical Chemistry, and I discussed my plans with Tak, as he was called. He had financed the construction of a bioscience center and had made that an integral part of his program. I also contacted the Midwest Research Institute in Kansas City, Missouri, where a few scientists were interested in the biochemistry of drugs. Now the only missing link was biology, and Tak came up with good idea: "Why don't we talk with Terry Johnson in Manhattan?"

Manhattan, fifty-six miles west of Lawrence, is the home of Kansas State University, the archrival of KU. Professor Johnson, chairman of the Department of Biology and Biochemistry, welcomed us with open arms, and it did not take long for the three of us to formulate an interactive program. Then the bomb exploded in the chancellor's office when Chancellor Dykes heard about it. Evidently the rivalry between the two universities extended beyond the playing fields—namely, into the budget of the state legislature. Dykes ordered Waxman to have a talk with Tak and me.

Waxman's office was not much bigger than ten by ten feet, and the walls were lined with chairs that did not normally belong there. Dave had called for a backup in the form of nine eagerly waiting chairmen of departments. The chairman of pharmacology and Kermit Kranz, the boss of OB-GYN, seemed to be licking their chops. I noticed the absence of Norton Greenberger, my chairman of medicine. Tak and I looked at each other, wondering what was going on, and we did not have to wait long to find out.

"I have heard rumors that you two have worked something out with the people in Manhattan behind my back," Waxman began. "The cancer center is part of the medical school and will stay right here."

"May I ask what you are talking about?" I asked.

"You know damn well what I am talking about. You and uh..." He pointed a finger at Tak, "Whatever your name is—you two plan to move the center to Lawrence and Manhattan."

Tak maintained his composure and dignity.

"Since when do you think that you can make the decisions around here?" Krantz wanted to know.

"I don't recall having to ask your permission for anything," I retorted.

However, it was clear that this was a gang killing, and Tak and I soon had enough and left.

"Sit down; I am not finished," Waxman ordered. We ignored him.

That was not the end of it. Dykes and Waxman began a campaign against me within the university and in the local press. They made false allegations, and I began to receive calls from the AP and UPI wanting my side of the story. I refused all interviews, and Tak also remained mum. Greenberger stayed out of it completely. Defending ourselves in the press would have been a losing battle, because in the State of Kansas people listened to the chancellor of the university, not two scientists. I called a meeting of the participants in the cancer program for the upcoming Friday in an effort to dispel the many wild stories. Members from all branches showed up, including people from Lawrence, and the amphitheater was packed. Kranz and his pharmacology stooge already occupied the center of the front row when I arrived. I was about to start, when an administrative assistant walked onstage and handed me an envelope. I put it in my pocket, explained where we stood with the center program, and said, "I'll answer questions if there are any."

Kermit Kranz could no longer control himself. "The letter—aren't you going to read the letter?"

"That's what you really came for, isn't it, Doctor Kranz? As if you do not already know what's in the letter."

It was a one-liner. "Ladies and gentlemen, I have been fired. Thank you for coming."

My crew insisted on taking me to Jimmy's for a beer; they had to vent their anger somehow.

"Why didn't that bastard Waxman hand you the letter?" Carol wanted to know.

"Because he is a coward—don't you understand?" Ron said, stating the obvious.

I went home after two beers and told Nienke what had happened.

"Does that mean that you're fired from the medical school?" she asked.

"No, I am a tenured professor and he can't touch that. But I am no longer director of the cancer center."

That night I thought back to the day that Waxman had said that I could not take his desk away from him. If only I had followed my intuition that day and walked out. I also should have resigned after I read that phony grant request. If another university had submitted a request like that, I would have voted against it in the study section. However, I had failed the university, and it was that failure that really hurt. I wasn't angry with Waxman; the man was nothing more than a flunky for Archie Dykes. Dykes had started it all. He had not been man enough to initiate a discussion with Tak and me. Tak was a huge international figure in his field, and Dykes remained ignorant of that fact.

The contact between the chancellor and I had been cordial up to then. In August 1976, I had written him a mildly critical letter. A joint Kansas House-Senate interim committee had held a public hearing about patient care at the medical center. A highly emotional woman addressed the committee saying that she was appalled by the poor physical condition of the hospital and the dirt. Several other speakers supported her. Over the years, she had made important contributions to KU, and she could not be ignored. The members of the committee did not know that her son was one of our patients, and I attempted to soften the overly harsh criticism. However, I agreed with her that there was room for improvement and urged the committee to pay attention to a renovation of the hospital in addition to adding a new building. A few other physicians and nurses also spoke up about the need for major revisions.

Following the hearing, Dykes told the press that the negative testimonies from a few dissatisfied persons did not trouble him. He called them "substantial exaggerations" coming from some staff members. However, he did admit that a long overdue, massive clean-up campaign would soon begin and that "the results should be highly visible within the next six months."

In a letter to Dykes, I expressed my disappointment that he had failed to support the excellent medical and nursing staff. "Do what you have to do for the outside world, but respect those who testified. They tried to help and cared enough to do so."

Three months later, he sent me a thank you note and a copy of a page in the program of the Kansas-Nebraska Football game. The page, complete with a photo of Cherri and me, featured the headquarters of SWOG and mentioned the millions of dollars in grant funds that the group brought to the university. "We appreciate the excellent work you are doing as a member of the faculty of the University of Kansas." In addition, a year later he thanked me for my talk during a luncheon with members of the legislature. "We could not have asked for a better representative of the medical center at this important luncheon." These letters were of the "Dear Barth" and the "Warmest wishes, Archie" type.

Why the sudden turnaround, and why didn't he let up after the "You are fired" letter? Dykes and Waxman continued their daily ad hominem attacks in the local press and on the radio. When the assistant manager of a radio station offered me time for rebuttal, I once more refused to comment. I wanted to keep that dirty laundry within the confines of the university. However, I did send a letter to Waxman, copied to the chancellor, in which I pointed out that their actions were hurting the university. "The university is more important than any of us, and, long after we are gone, the university will continue to be a center for higher education." I offered to discuss the matter in private and hoped that a joint press release would conclude the controversy. Waxman's secretary called to say that a meeting was set up for the following Saturday morning in the office of the senior executive vice-chancellor.

Dykes did not show up. Instead, there was Waxman and his entourage of chairmen, led by Kranz. I stayed in the hallway.

"Come on in, Barth," Waxman said from behind his desk.

"No, you come out, alone."

"Oh don't be childish. Come in."

"You either come out or there will be no meeting."

There followed a murmur of voices, and then, one by one, they filed out past me; Kranz, with a screwy smile, was last.

"Now will you come in?"

"No, you come out, and we'll meet in the conference room."

I knew better not to meet with him sitting behind his desk. Dean Lowman joined us in the conference room. The door closed, and I exploded, calling Waxman a coward, a stooge, a lowdown nothing, and an assortment of other choice epithets. He actually went down on one knee and begged me. "I'm sorry. I really am sorry. I just did what I was told to do. I'll do anything, anything. Tell me what you want, and I'll do it," he said in a trembling voice.

"I want you to get someone in here to write a letter."

That someone turned out to be an assistant dean. I dictated the letter stating that Dr. Waxman and I had reached an agreement to immediately discontinue all adversarial press releases and that for the good of the university the matter regarding the cancer center was closed. We sat in awkward silence while waiting for the assistant dean to bring in the letter and four copies.

"Now sign it," I said to Waxman.

"I can't. I must show it to Dykes first."

"Damn it, you are going back on your word."

"I will sign the letter. You will have it Monday. I'll bring you a signed copy. I swear, as God is my witness."

"Dave, you know what will happen if I don't have that signed copy by Monday, don't you?"

I went home emotionally exhausted. I parked the car at the side of the road and waited for my legs to stop trembling. A good cry would have helped, but the tears did not come. It took a while before I managed a wry smile, and when I drove on, it felt like a heavy load had been lifted off me.

The signed copy was delivered on Monday. Dykes did not last long as chancellor; he went to an insurance company where he did not last either. Waxman was shuttled aside not long after that. However, before Dykes left, there was a sequel to the affair.

Three of our children are KU graduates. "Dad, all students who graduate first in their class received a commendation letter from Chancellor Dykes during the graduation ceremony. I was first twice and he didn't give me any." Evelien was close to tears when she told me this. Archie Dykes had shown how small a man he really was, and I fired off a letter. "No matter what went on between you and me, I remind you that you are still the head of a teaching institution of which our daughter was a student. You forgot your responsibility as a teacher and have hurt our daughter. I trust that you will rectify your error immediately." Three days later Evelien received two signed commendation letters from him.

22

BECOMING A REAL DOCTOR AGAIN

Nienke and I talked it over, and we decided that it was time to leave Kansas. I could take the treatment by Dykes and Waxman, but I could not forget the total lack of support from my chairman during the ugly episode. I had no trouble giving up the chair of SWOG. After nine years, it was time for a change in leadership that would bring fresh energy and new ideas for growth. A third factor was my experience during the sabbatical, and Nienke pointed it out to me. "You really liked being with patients while we were in Cairo. You were different then, and you talked about your work with them. Remember, you said that you felt like a doctor again?"

She was right; I had enjoyed the interaction with patients and colleagues. Maybe I could return to a practice. Nienke had her own reason for making a change. The nest was empty. Frank had a challenging job in a television station and wanted to stay in Kansas. Evelien would soon graduate from the music conservatory and begin working. Marion had asked me what she should major in after she came back from Egypt. "I thought of Arabic, Dad, but they only teach classical Arabic in colleges, and that has no practical use."

"Study Chinese. There are more than a billion people in China. They are hard working and smart, and they are not going to be under the control of the communists forever."

Marion became fluent in speaking, reading, and writing Chinese, and after she graduated, she was one of four Americans selected as exchange students. She lived in Beijing with a Chinese roommate and roamed around the country. This was not permitted, but when caught she always managed to talk her way out of it largely because the officials had never met a blond American woman who spoke their tongue. When her year was nearly finished, Nienke wrote her a letter. "Don't you dare fly back. Find another way to travel and see the world. I will send Nick over so that you two can travel together." They made the long, adventurous trip from Beijing on the Trans-Siberian Railroad, around Lake Baikal, and through Siberia to Moscow. Then they traveled through communist Poland via Warsaw and East Germany to Berlin, where they entered the world of luxury and had their first good meal in weeks.

Marion was now in Yale's Law School, and Nick also decided to become a lawyer. It was time for me to make some money. It was on a Friday in January 1981, at about 6:00 PM that I returned to the SWOG office and saw a note on my desk. "Call Bethesda."

"What would the NCI want so late?" I wondered, but while I dialed the number I saw that it was not the Washington area code." A man answered.

"Dr. Hoogstraten, my name is Tom Wilburn, and I am the director of Bethesda Hospital. We are building a cancer treatment center and—"

"Excuse me for interrupting, sir, but where is your hospital?"

"Oh, I'm sorry. We're in Cincinnati, Ohio."

"Thank you."

"Well, we are looking for a director for the center, and I have been told that you are in a position to make some recommendations."

"Mr. Wilburn, I get many requests like that, and I am sorry, but unless you give me some details, I will not recommend anybody."

"I understand. Bethesda has two hospitals with the largest patient population in the city." He proceeded to paint a nice picture of Cincinnati and the hospital, and while he was talking I began to think "Why not me?"

"We want to open the center on July 1, and I hope to have someone aboard by that time."

"Sir, you sound like a good salesman to me. So good that as a matter of fact I may be interested."

"That is more than I expected. Would you mind paying us a visit?'

"Can I bring my wife along?"

"By all means do." We arranged for a visit early in February.

"How would you like to go to Cincinnati?" I said, surprising Nienke when I came home.

"When?" She was always game to go wherever life took us.

The telephone call had made up my mind; we were leaving Kansas. On Monday, I called Chuck Coltman in San Antonio.

"Chuck, I am going to resign as chairman of SWOG, and I would like nothing better than if you were to succeed me."

"That's a surprise. How did that come about?"

"Never mind how, but I will officially announce it at the next meeting. I just wanted you to know so that you can do your homework. You can keep it under your hat or do anything you want, but be prepared for an election."

I knew that Chuck not only wanted to become chairman but also that he would be the best man for the job. At the meeting in April, I made the announcement, called a meeting of the principal investigators, and asked for candidates. Sid Salmon from Tucson nominated Coltman, and Freireich nominated himself with a long speech explaining why he was the only legitimate candidate. Coltman received all but three votes. I congratulated him, resigned as a member of SWOG, and left. Several members called me afterwards. "Barth, why did you resign from the group?"

"Because, Chuck should not have someone looking over his shoulder, and this way nobody can complain to me about the changes that he is going to make."

The old SWOG members of the new pediatric oncology group gave me a set of golf clubs and a series of lessons. The adult members presented me with a gold coin, a Krugerrand. I had no idea where the thing had disappeared to until Nienke reminded me that she had put it in our safety deposit box.

Doctors' wives pleasantly entertained Nienke during our first visit to Cincinnati. While I was brushing my teeth before going to bed, she gave me an enthusiastic report of the beauty of the city and its suburbs. Tom Wilburn and members of the Bethesda Hospital staff told me all there was to know about the hospital and medical community. Tom wanted me to meet the chairman of the board, who was also chairman of the board of the Kroger Company. We would meet him for lunch at the Kenwood Country Club, and, as we drove on Kenwood Road, Tom slowed down and pointed to a house standing two hundred feet back from the road. "There's your house, Barth, it just came on the market."

The chairman, a robust man in his seventies, insisted that I call him Jake, "Because everybody does." He was there to give me a good looking over and asked some sharp questions. "What is the state of the art in cancer therapy in Cincinnati?"

"It is not up to par with other large cities by a long shot."

"Why not?"

"The medical school isn't exactly known for its cancer research program, and the city as a whole seems to be a wasteland as far as cancer is concerned. Nothing stands out, except of course the children's hospital."

"What about the incidence of cancer? Cincinnati has a very high incidence according to the newspaper reports"

"I have no opinion about that until I have seen the report."

Wilburn had remained silent, but on the way back he explained why Bethesda wanted its own cancer treatment center. "Jake is Mr. Cincinnati, and he and his friends have not been happy with the cancer programs in the city for quite some years. They are very disturbed about the report of the high incidence of cancer for which the author blames industrial pollution."

"Who prepared that report?"

"A professor in the medical school—a statistician, I think."

We had a preliminary discussion about the salary for the director for the cancer treatment center and the other benefits, and Wilburn mentioned that the appointment needed the approval of the medical staff. Nienke and I looked at the house on Kenwood Road, but she did not want it. "The house is too small, and the yard is too big." It was two and a half acres with about sixty trees, a swimming pool, and a tennis court. We left Wilburn with the impression that we were interested, although I had some reservations about my benefits, and I wanted a guaranteed income for two years, during which I could develop a practice. Three months later, he flew to Kansas City with a contract that still had a few blanks. After lunch we sat down on our porch, he agreed to my conditions, filled in the blanks, and we signed. Once more, I sat for a state medical licensing examination.

Instead of immediately buying a house, we decided to rent for a few months so that Nienke could look around. I made a third trip to Cincinnati, bought a copy of the *Cincinnati Enquirer*, and looked for houses for rent. All owners wanted a deposit and a contract for a year. The last house was on Avery Lane where it dead-ends on Observatory Park. It was much too small and had only a tiny one-car garage. I had one last look and walked to my car.

"Yoo-hoo." A lady came running across the street. "Are you interested in renting that house?"

"Not really. It's too small. We would have to store most of our furniture."

"Oh, that's no problem; we have lots of space in our house. Come, we'll talk about it."

Her name was Carolyn, and she lived in the large rambling house across the street where her parents had lived and where she was born. "This is my husband John Caldwell. Now what would you like to drink?"

John was an easygoing, loose-limbed man who talked with a laugh in his voice. They were our age. He was proud of his Kentucky-Appalachian background, and he was the ombudsman of the *Cincinnati Enquirer*. Like all newspaper people, he enjoyed a hearty drink, and it was about that time. "Never mind the lemonade, Carolyn; perhaps the doctor likes a real drink?"

We asked about our backgrounds, and one could not imagine meeting two friendlier people.

"For how long do you want to rent?" Carolyn had already decided that I would take that little house.

"I don't know. Long enough for Nienke to make up her mind. Three, four months I guess."

"Great. Is the price all right?"

"That's fine. Do you want a deposit now?"

"Oh we don't bother about a deposit or a contract. You just stay as long as you like—until you buy a house."

Soon after coming to Cincinnati, the city council held an open meeting to discuss the high rate of cancer ("The highest incidence of any town in the country"). The secretary of the chamber of commerce asked me to attend. The mayor gave a short introduction and then invited citizens to come forward and address their concerns. Several people had an opinion, and a number of them were highly emotional about it. Then the mayor called on the professor from the university who had written the report. He essentially confirmed what the press had already printed. The mayor thanked him, leaned forward to the microphone, and asked, "Is Dr. Hoogstraten in the audience?"

"Yes sir, I am."

"Would you mind saying a few words, doctor?"

I pointed out that not every hospital in the city reported its new cancer patients to a central tumor registry, and I therefore questioned the reliability of the data from which the professor had drawn his conclusions. I also noted that the professor had failed to make an adjustment for age when he calculated the incidence of cancer.

"Cincinnati is a beautiful city, and most people love to stay here after they retire. We know that the incidence of cancer increases significantly as people get older, so I would not be surprised if, relatively speaking, there were more cancer patients in Cincinnati than in other cities. However, we have no right to compare our city with other cities until the age factor has been included in the calculations. We must also take into account that about half of our population is of German stock, and I wonder whether that influences the incidence. So instead of being prematurely concerned about an unproven high incidence of cancer, I urge the professor to have another look at the data."

While talking, I maintained eye contact with the mayor and the two women on the council.

"Thank you, Doctor. Council was not previously informed about the importance of age."

The chamber of commerce breathed easier after the meeting, and journalists from both papers asked me questions afterwards.

"What are your thoughts about the quality of cancer care in Cincinnati, Doctor?"

"It could be better."

"You mind expanding on that?"

"Take, for instance, radiation therapy. There are four large hospitals and a medical school, and there is not a single linear accelerator in the entire city. That means that some of the radiotherapy is outdated. In addition, the city has very few CAT scanners to detect whether the cancer has spread. A hospital without a CAT scanner is not up-to-date these days." These and some other comments made the front page the next day.

My new secretary buzzed, "Doctor Aron is on the phone for you."

"Barth, remember me? You and I were in Beth-El together."

"Bernie, good to hear your voice. Where are you?"

"Here—in Cincinnati—and I want to thank you for your comment about the linear accelerator. I have been trying to get one for years, but the medical school is dragging its feet. Maybe now they'll do something about it."

Bernie had studied radiation therapy at Mount Sinai, and he was now the chairman of the radiation therapy department at the university here. Dr. Harry Horwitz, the director of Oncologists Associates, the most dominant oncology group in the city, was not so happy. In the next day's newspapers, he declared: "Our patients receive just as good radiation with the Cobalt machine." If that were true, why did all major hospitals within two years obtain an accelerator, and why did he use them so much?

Betty

It didn't take long before I had a thriving private practice, and I had to admit that taking care of patients full-time was quite different from making the rounds as a professor in a medical school and having the fellows and residents take over after rounds. I knew my chemotherapy, but I was rusty in the day-to-day department. However, it was fun, and I felt like a doctor again even if the phone rang at night. One of my first patients was Betty, a good-looking forty-five-year-old with an infectious smile. She was well read, a good golfer, and she had a loving family. She had cancer of the ovary, and, as was unfortunately the case in most patients with that disease, it had already spread throughout the abdomen at the time of her diagnosis.

"Mrs. H…?"

"Please call me Betty," she interrupted.

"Thank you. Tell me what you have learned so far about your condition."

"I know that I have cancer of the ovary and that it has spread," she said calmly.

"You know also that I am a medical oncologist."

"Yes, I do."

"And what do you think that means?"

She hesitated a moment. "I think it means that there is no cure." Her lips pressed together. I let my hand rest on her shoulder.

"It means that I cannot promise you anything, except that I'll take good care of you," I said with a faint smile.

"I know you will."

"Let's first see how you do on Melphalan. It is a small pill, and it will not make you sick, I promise."

"That is something, isn't it?" It was her turn for a faint smile.

Unlike my mentor, Louis Wasserman, who never told his patients the diagnosis or the progress of the disease, I am a firm believer in maintaining a frank dialogue with patients. Doctors can be sensitive to the needs of their patients and still tell it as it is. "Never underestimate their capacity to absorb bad news," I taught my students. "And always have a warm feeling for them."

Betty usually came with her mother, a charming, petite, silver-haired lady. I never did meet her husband. Moreover, she did respond to the Melphalan. Today's oncologists may scoff at its use, but thirty years ago, we did not have much else. She went back to playing golf and lived a good life for eight months, when the cancer cells became resistant to the drug and multiplied as never before. Two other drugs failed.

"Betty, I can do no more for you except make you as comfortable as possible. Have you thought where you want to be when the end comes?"

"I'd like to be at home." Her calmness made my task easy.

"I'll make some arrangement, and now I'll say good bye."

"Thank you for all you did," she said.

As I turned to the door, she called me back. "Doctor, please give me a kiss?"

So we kissed. Three weeks later, I read in the newspaper that she had died, and nine months thereafter her mother stopped me in the hallway. "When can I get my baby back?"

"What do you mean?"

"She gave her body to the university, but it has been long enough. Can you please find out?"

I called the medical school, and they released the body that same day.

Years later, when I had already retired, I thought of Betty when a dear friend was in the terminal phase of her colon cancer. She had a terrific sense of humor and at Halloween parties always showed up with an outrageous costume. We roared when she came one year in a flesh-colored body leotard on which certain body parts were clearly outlined.

"I have never died before," she said to me one day. "Can you tell me something about it? Are there any good books."

"If I tell you that there is nothing to dying, I would be stretching the truth a bit, but I do know that you will do fine." We talked for fifteen minutes and parted with a hug.

"One of her last requests was to thank you," her husband said after the funeral. "I didn't know you two had talked. She was calm and clear-minded to the end."

Tom

A World War II veteran was just as clear-minded when he died. Tom was a tough man. During the war, he served in the navy shipyards working on torpedo boats and light cruisers. He was a bachelor, until he met a widow with a two-year-old boy, Tommy. Tom, then forty-eight years old, loved Tommy, and it was not long before he married Tommy's mother. He was a heavy smoker, and, like all smokers, he had developed a chronic cough. His chest X-rays showed a marked thickening of the lining of his left lung, and a biopsy revealed a mesothelioma. The risk of developing a mesothelioma is between one hundred and one thousand times higher in asbestos workers than in the general population, and Tom was a victim of asbestos as well as cigarettes.

After I told him the diagnosis, he immediately contacted a lawyer and found out that the State of California expedited lawsuits involving cancer caused by prolonged exposure to asbestos. Tom became a client of a San Francisco law firm that specialized in asbestosis, waited, and waited some more while his condition worsened. Finally, I wrote his lawyer that I could not expect Tom to live more that three or four months. Two months later, the lawyer called. Tom's suit was scheduled in court in ten days, and he wanted Tom to fly to California.

"There's no way he can fly. He is tied to an oxygen tank," I told him.

"Then his wife and son must be in the courtroom when the judge hears the case."

Tom convinced his wife to go to California and take Tommy with her. "Doc, you got to keep me alive until this is settled," he said.

Alone, Tom went downhill fast. He entered the hospital and ten days later transferred to the intensive care unit (ICU). There was still no news from California. Tom went on life support and held on. My phone rang. It was the lawyer. "Doctor, we won the case, and the company has settled for a lot of money."

I went to the ICU. "Tom, you won big. Your family will be taken care of."

"That's all I wanted," Tom whispered. "Now cut the juice."

"Cut the juice?" I did not get it immediately.

"Just let me go. Pull the plug."

I pulled the plug and stayed with Tom while he died.

Esther

Nothing pleases an oncologist more than a patient who survives against overwhelming odds. Esther beat the odds. She had melanoma, which is the worst possible malignancy of the skin. She had noticed a change of color in a mole on her right lower leg and it turned out to be melanoma. The surgeon made a wide excision around the tumor and the edges of the excised tissue were free of tumor cells. Nineteen months later, she felt a swelling in her groin, and the same surgeon removed all lymph nodes in that area. Two nodes contained melanoma cells. Nearly two years later Esther showed up in my office with a pitch-black tumor the size of a quarter in the same area. A small piece of the tumor was missing.

"Who did that?" I asked.

"My surgeon took a piece again," she said.

Why remove a piece if you already know the obvious diagnosis? The black tumor was just the tip of the iceberg, because beneath was a mass as big as my fist firmly fixed to the underlying tissue. The rest of her physical examination was negative, as were her chest X-rays. Now what? Esther was an intelligent woman, and she knew that it was serious.

"I can give you combination chemotherapy, but you should know that only about one in ten patients respond, and usually it is only a partial response."

"Anything else we can do?" she asked. "What about surgery or radiation?"

"The tumor has infiltrated into the deep tissue, and I doubt that any surgeon will advise you to have another operation, and unfortunately melanoma is practically resistant to radiation."

"Then it has to be chemotherapy, and we might as well start now." Her mind was made up, and I really thought that she already had decided on chemotherapy before she came to see me. Esther not only responded, the tumor melted away in record time. After four courses of combination chemotherapy, the tumor was no longer palpable, and after six the underlying tissue that had been as hard as a rock was smooth and soft.

"I have never seen anything like it," I confessed.

"Will it stay away?" she asked.

"I don't know, but in the meantime you can count your blessings."

I had no idea why she had responded. Was it the result of the chemotherapy or had the surgeon evoked some immunologic effect when he cut into the tumor? The melanoma did stay away; at least, it did not recur in the nine years that I saw Esther. She loved to crochet and made two large blankets for us, which after twenty-five years we still use.

Esther and Chuck, the patient in Kansas with the huge inoperable tumor in his abdomen, are cured of their disease. Are they true miracles? And what about John with his terminal myeloma? Physicians do not believe in miracles, least of all the oncologists, and yet many of us have observed seemingly unexplainable "cures" in our practice. Although we do not like to use the word *miracle*, we are sometimes at a loss for a better word. Experiences such as those of Chuck and Esther do not stay long within the confines of family and friends. People love to talk about the unusual and like the phrase *miracles will happen*. Patients, family members, friends, and—yes—doctors continue to use that term. "There is always hope, isn't there, doctor?"

Yes, there is, and it is not unusual for a doctor to reply, "You never know. A miracle may happen."

Louise

Unfortunately, I also witnessed an ugly situation. Louise was a sweet, elderly black woman with metastatic breast cancer. The disease had spread to several bones, and her main complaint was severe pain. During every visit to the clinic, she had her doting son at her side. He pushed her wheelchair into the examining room, helped her onto the table, assisted with the removal of clothing, gently took her arms, guided them into the sleeves of a gown, and then he took a seat on a chair.

"Hello Louise, how are you doing today?" I would ask when I entered the room.

"Momma has a lot of pain doctor," the son would reply. "A lot of pain."

Louise never said much, and on the few occasions when she started to say something, her son would inevitably interrupt. "I'm with her all day doctor. I know how much Momma suffers."

Two months later he said, "We have to see you more often doctor. Momma's pain pills do not last as long as they once did."

"Well, let's take at new bone scan and look at the X-rays first," I said. The repeat photos showed the same amount of bone involvement and no appreciable change in the old lesions.

"How much pain do you have Louise?" I asked during her next visit.

"It's getting—" began the son.

I cut him off. "No, you be quiet. I want your mother to answer me."

Louise's face, which usually bore a faint smile, changed to uncertainty, and then a fright came in her eyes. I turned around just in time to see the son glower at her with tight jaws and a warning, fixed stare. His face immediately relaxed, and he smiled warmly at Momma when he saw me looking.

"You get out of the room," I ordered the son, but I had not been fast enough, because Louise had already clammed up. There was nothing left to do other than write her a new prescription and give her another appointment. That same afternoon a suburban pharmacist called me, "Doctor, I have your prescription for Percocet for Mrs. A. Do you know that she also goes to the clinic here?"

"No, I was under the impression that she was only being seen by me."

"Well, her son brought your prescription in yesterday and two days ago he had one from our clinic."

"Thanks for bringing that to my attention. Do me a favor; do not fill my prescription. Make some excuse. Can you do that?"

"Sure, and will you take care of it?"

"I will." I contacted the police and a few days later an officer came to see me. "That son of a bitch had his mother in four clinics. He collected the pills and sold them on the street. His mother never got a single pill."

The doting son was packed off in jail. Louise continued to see me, but now a friendly member of her church accompanied her and saw to it that she received her pain medication. I wonder how often this has happened in other families.

Sylvia

A "cancer" that is not a true cancer can present a dilemma for the oncologist. A middle-aged woman called for an appointment, and my secretary instructed her to bring the operating report with her, the X-rays, a copy of the pathology report, and the tissue slides from which the diagnosis was made. I examined her, and, except for a well-healed scar of a modified radical mastectomy, there was nothing unusual in the rest of my examination.

"Did you feel the tumor yourself?" I asked Sylvia.

"It was right here," she pointed to a spot on her other breast. "It started out as a pimple, and it gradually became an ulcer."

As a pimple?

The pre-op note read, "Surgery for inflammatory breast cancer with ulceration."

The physical appearance of inflammatory breast cancer is usually sufficient for the diagnosis. The skin is reddish and has the appearance and consistency of an orange peel. We use the French term *peau d'orange* to describe it. We do not recommend a biopsy because most patients already have signs of advanced cancer involving many lymph nodes and distant spread. The treatment in eight renowned institutions has consisted of chemotherapy, followed by radiation therapy. In four institutions the patients then had a simple mastectomy, but only if there was no evidence of disease after the initial therapy. The surgery did not make any difference. None of 376 patients initially had a mastectomy, and surgery has been discarded as the primary therapy for this presentation of cancer of the breast.

Sylvia's surgeon in her small town in northern Ohio was probably not familiar with these reports. They all came out between 1980 and 1986. When I looked at the pathology slides, I saw no evidence of breast cancer and neither did our pathologist. Now what was I to tell the patient? That she never had breast cancer and should not have had the mastectomy? That she only had an infection? She did not come to see me to hear that. She wanted to know what to do next, if anything. If I told her the truth, she would be miserable for the rest of her life and agonize about her deformity every time she looked into the mirror. Eventually the people in her town would hear about it, and then what?

"Sylvia, you are one of the luckiest women I've seen in my practice. You are free of cancer, and you don't need any chemotherapy or other form of treatment."

"That makes me so happy to hear. Thank you so much, doctor."

Was I wrong in not telling her the truth? When I addressed that question to several colleagues during a meeting, most agreed with the way I had handled the situation. However, there were a few who hesitated with "Maybe there was a way of somehow letting her know." However, when I asked them how, they could not tell. A young doctor said, "I would have no trouble telling her the truth. Surgeons like that have no business operating on patients. She can sue the man." That one doctor was too hard-nosed for me. He worked in a large cancer institute and had no idea how physicians in the small towns throughout America practice, how intensely the people interact with their doctor. They see them in church, in meetings, and at parties, and they trust their doctor, because he is the best. However, I did have a telephone conversation with the doctor.

Hector

My greatest success as a doctor came in 1964 with an unemployed carpenter from the Dominican Republic who was a frequent patient on the medical floors. Hector's main complaints were weakness, a slight fever, and vague pain in the right upper abdomen. He had exploratory surgery twice, but nothing was found. I had to see a patient on his floor and went to Hector's bed by mistake. His story intrigued me, and I asked his resident for a sample of his blood, which showed a distinct abnormality in his serum protein. His bone marrow contained no abnormal plasma cells, his urine was normal, and X-rays showed no skeletal lesions. What could be wrong with him?

Chronic irritation in the abdomen of a mouse can lead to an abnormal accumulation of plasma cells, and I wondered whether Hector could have a chronic infection somewhere in his abdomen.

"Hector, I just have an inkling about the cause of your trouble, and I'd like to see whether one of my drugs can help you."

"What kind of drug, doctor?"

"It is called Melphalan, and it is used in patients with a rare form of cancer."

"Cancer? Do I have cancer?"

"No, you don't. But I found an abnormality in your blood that is also seen in that rare cancer and with Melphalan the abnormality sometimes disappears."

"Will it make me sick?"

"No, but I'll have to keep an eye on your blood count."

"Well, nothing else has helped doctor. I'll try it."

Hector received Melphalan for three months as an outpatient, and gradually the serum spike disappeared. The three months was also the longest time he had been without symptoms. I saw him every three months thereafter, and then Christmas rolled around.

"There is a package for you in your office," my secretary said when I returned from making rounds one December day.

Some package. It was a box with six bottles of my favorite single-malt Scotch. There was no card with the box. Who on Earth had given me such an expensive present in a city hospital like Elmhurst? Nearly all our patients were on Welfare or Medicaid; surely none could afford a present like that.

"Who brought this?" I asked Terry.

"A driver in uniform. I think he was a chauffeur."

Ah. That was it. A wealthy Mount Sinai patient must have sent it. Nevertheless, why no name? Around eleven o'clock my door opened and a smiling Hector walked in.

"Is that the right Scotch?" he asked.

"Hector—you?"

"Yes sir."

Hector was fashionably dressed, unlike the unemployed carpenter I knew.

"What's going on? And what's with the chauffeur?"

"Well doctor, you are looking at the ambassador of the Dominican Republic to the United Nations."

"You're kidding me."

"It's true. My school buddy became the president of my country, and he appointed me as the new ambassador."

"Your school buddy?"

"Yes, President Balaguer is my friend."

And so it happened that I treated an unemployed carpenter who then became an ambassador. The next Christmas Hector brought another six-pack of Scotch, and he came to say good-bye four months thereafter. He and his brother had bought a factory in the Dominican Republic and they were going to make doors. In the July 15, 2002, issue of *The New York Times* I read the obituary of Joaquin Balaguer, and I wondered what had happened to Hector, my greatest success story.

ASCO—Just an opinion

I am not pleased with the direction clinical oncology has taken. The American Society of Clinical Oncology (ASCO) has grown enormously over the thirty-nine years since its inception, and, if numbers alone are a measure of success, then the society has been a success indeed. I remember the first meeting in 1964 when the attendance was about one hundred and fifty. In 2003 the membership had grown to over twenty thousand, and twenty-five thousand people attended the annual meeting. The criteria for active membership are vague, and less than half of the members are board certified in medical oncology.

The proceedings of the 2003 meeting, printed in a book of 11,061 pages, contained 3,641 abstracts, the vast majority of which remained unread. They were replete with reports of studies that only contained so-called preliminary results and, as such, had little or no value.

ASCO shows no discrimination and little judgment when it comes to printing abstracts such as the one submitted by the authors from the Albert Einstein College of Medicine, who studied the effect of yoga on the quality of life of the cancer patient (Abstract 2921). The authors concluded that preliminary results appear to show that yoga may act as a buffer to the physical, emotional, and social symptoms associated with breast cancer and its treatment. That should surprise nobody. The NCI paid for that study. The people at the Mayo Clinic went a step or two further when they compared a group of patients that received normal cancer care with a group that was entertained, as well as cared for by a large team comprising a psychiatrist, a psychologist, chaplains, social workers, physical therapists, and nurses (Abstract 2925). They called this "structured multidisciplinary psychosocial intervention," and guess what? The entertainers stated that they gave patients a better quality of life. The children in a kindergarten class could have told them that.

A group of seven physicians at the Memorial Sloan-Kettering Cancer Center must have been bored. They could not come up with any good ideas, so they decided to study the obvious. They went through the records of 1,405 patients to see whether patients who had a drop in their blood count after a first course of chemotherapy had more severe toxicity after subsequent courses than patients whose count had not dropped. We knew that forty years ago, but it is reassuring to know that today's chemotherapists notice the same obvious phenomenon.

The NCI, Weight-Watchers, and the Ford Motor Company Fund supported a study of weight and depression in a small group of forty-eight obese breast cancer survivors. Six investigators at Wayne State University in Detroit start off by writing, "Obese breast cancer survivors *may have* [emphasis added] shortened recurrence-free survival." An effective weight loss strategy is *thus* a priority, they claim. However, what if the "may have" is not true? Should they not first have given evidence for their premise? They divided their patients into four mini-groups of twelve patients and approached each group with a different strategy. These mini-groups were too small to detect significant differences, so when the authors analyzed the results, they put two groups together. Their conclusions contain words such as *likely* and *may*, and just maybe they did not have enough patients to do the study.

Why does ASCO continue to print thousands of abstracts indiscriminately, without any screening at all? Where is the science in that? Moreover, what is the use of sending out the abstracts several weeks after the meeting? Is that not an admission that they are essentially useless? ASCO, where is your pride?

The Pharmaceutical Industry: A New Cancer?

I believe that a new cancer has infiltrated the ranks of oncologists, a cancer called the pharmaceutical industry. I first learned of this cancer in 1982 when Adria Laboratories asked me to participate in a study comparing its highly effective anticancer drug Adriamycin with a slight variant of that drug. The company would reimburse me for my costs, and I saw no harm in that. The trouble began when at the end of the study, the company announced that its own statisticians would analyze and report the results. This of course created the possibility of bias in favor of one drug over the other, and I vehemently objected. When the company insisted, I refused to have my name used as a co-author. Later, a colleague pointed out to me that I had been naïve. "Didn't you know that their patent for Adriamycin was running out and that they needed the variant to keep going?" The thought had never entered my mind.

My second encounter came when Bristol-Myers wanted to compare Megace—a compound derived from the hormone progesterone—with Tamoxifen—an antiestrogen that was a big winner in the treatment of primary breast cancer and patients with advanced disease. Years earlier, we had given Megace to a few women with advanced breast cancer, and it did have some benefit: namely, increased appetite and weight gain. Bristol-Myers had obtained the rights to Megace and wanted a piece of the pie. I helped with the writing of the protocol, and, since X-rays were going to be the most important determinant for the evaluation of the results, I insisted that Bob Talley of the Henry Ford Hospital in Detroit and I review all X-rays, without payment. The company agreed, and the study began.

Imagine my surprise when I received a telegram from Bristol-Myers eight months later announcing that they would submit an abstract of the study to ASCO before the deadline, which was three days later. They faxed an abstract to me, and I had two hours to call in suggestions for 'minor' changes. The first author was a hotshot who at that time claimed to be the youngest chairman of medicine in the country. He had not entered any patients in the study; in other words, he was a ghostwriter, a patsy for Bristol-Myers. He had not seen any of the X-rays. I called in a minor change—"Remove my name from the abstract." The abstract described only the protocol; there were no results, and the last sentence read, "Preliminary results, to be presented, indicate that Megace may have comparable efficacy in breast cancer." ASCO accepted the abstract.

The study continued, and some time later, the ghostwriter wrote an article with himself as the first author. He added Bob Talley and me as co-authors. Company statisticians had analyzed the study, Bob and I had not seen all the X-rays, and the author considered Megace just as good as Tamoxifen and recommended it as an alternate first-line drug for metastatic cancer. I fired off a letter to Dr. Stephen Carter at Bristol-Myers to object to the misuse of data to reach an invalid conclusion and a misleading recommendation, and I again insisted on the removal of my name. Carter did not respond and Megace died on the vine; today it is only recommended for patients with AIDS who have significant weight loss.

Pharmaceutical giant Pfizer pulled a similar stunt in the 1990s when the company supported a study comparing its Fluconazole with Amphotericin B, made by Bristol-Myers. Both drugs were used to prevent fungal infection, but Fluconazole was new, and Pfizer wanted a share of the market. The company provided the drugs, gave financial assistance to the investigators, and performed the statistical analyses. Few people should be surprised that when the results were published in the *Journal of the American Medical Association* (*JAMA*), Fluconazole turned out to be the better drug. However, two Danish investigators learned that Pfizer had used amphotericin B given by mouth instead of intravenously. That was dirty pool because Pfizer already knew that oral amphotericin B was ineffective. Both Pfizer and the *JAMA* refused to comment when the Danes contacted them.

Drug companies have found other ways to influence the outcomes of studies. During the last five years or so, they have appointed numerous oncologists as "consultants," and pay them fees for their service. They also found a need for them on their boards of directors and on company advisory committees. Quite a number of researchers use the words "employed by" to describe their connection with drug companies while at the same time they are fully employed by their university. The infiltration is so widespread that most reputable journals now require that all authors complete a disclosure statement about their ties to the drug industry during the preceding two years.

ASCO demonstrated just how bad this has become by adding 999 pages to its 2003 Proceedings, because the authors of all 3,641 abstracts had to provide the information. No less than 975, or 26.8 percent of the authors, served as consultant, advisor, and/or on the boards of companies. Of the first 1,000 abstracts listed in the Proceedings, 483 researchers, or 48.3 percent, had financial ties to drug companies, which ASCO defines as "honoraria in excess of $2,000 per year or $ 5,000 over a three-year period." However, the society's definition leaves room for far higher honoraria. The champion with the longest disclosure list was ASCO President Dr. Paul A. Bunn, Jr., a consultant to nine drug companies. He received a grant from one of them and holds stock in a privately held company. During the May 2002 meeting of ASCO, Dr. Bunn told reporters that the results of the experimental drug Iressa "seem better than one would get with standard chemotherapy." Did Bunn also mention that he received an honorarium from AstraZeneca, the company that produces Iressa?

Unfortunately, there is no reason to believe that cancer researchers are the only ones with the dubious honor of being a paid consultant, board member, or advisor. Other medical specialties are likely to be equally infiltrated by the pharmaceutical industry. At an August 2000 meeting of the Department of Health and Human Services, Dr. Jane Henney, the commissioner of the Food and Drug Administration, questioned whether researchers with financial ties to drug companies gave unbiased evaluations of their data. The problem gets worse when companies such as Bristol-Myers hire well-known researchers to do the dirty job as a so-called "guest author" for studies that they had not conducted or in which they had not participated. In 1996, Dr. Thomas Bodenheimer of the University of California at San Francisco reported that of 809 articles published in six major medical journals, no less than twenty-nine percent had guest authors and/or ghostwriters. There is no doubt in my mind that these drug companies introduce bias in favor of their products.

"Why do you want to retire? You still have so much to give," Dr. Dieter Hossfeld said over lunch in 1991 in Hamburg, Germany. "You are still so young."

"Dieter, I am sixty-seven, and I don't want to flame-out."

"Flame-out? What does that mean, Barth?"

"It means that I don't want to hang on to the bitter end. Besides, I want to start a new part of my life." I decided to stop when I could no longer satisfactorily answer the questions posed by the fellows and residents. I could not keep up with the literature and with the rapid new developments. Moreover, frankly, it was because I was no longer was enthusiastic about my work.

There were other considerations. Our children were married, and we had a bunch of grandchildren. I wanted to stay home and share good times with Nienke. She had never complained through the years when I was too busy to give her my undivided attention. This was now our golden time when we could enjoy each other's company and do so many things together. I had never realized how nice that could be. I am now the official vacuum man of the house; I set the table for breakfast and dinner, and help with the dishes…sometimes. I am also the official salad maker. We live on Daufuskie Island, a five by two and a half mile oasis off the coast of South Carolina, with no cars, no shops, a small First Baptist church, and a two-room schoolhouse for twenty-four students. Magnificent trees surround us. We have beaches, pitch-dark skies at night with the brightest stars, and silence, beautiful silence. There are birds, deer, alligators, raccoons, fish, and no skunks. We ride our bikes, swim, walk, travel, and I play golf two times a week. In addition, we helped build a museum. Now that is living!

I keep in contact with friends and former colleagues and now and then go to a meeting of ASCO or ASH, the American Society of Hematology. Last year ASH gave me a clock with a plaque stating that I was a distinguished emeritus member of ASH. I did not know there was such a category of membership, but I appreciated the nice gesture and went to the December meeting in Philadelphia. My friend Dr. Dorothea Zucker-Franklin asked me to be her escort to a reception for the past-presidents of the society and it was great fun to see my old friends. In 1958, I was privileged when Lou Wasserman took me to Boston where Dr. Louis Diamond, a professor of pediatrics, presided over one of the organizing meetings of ASH, and I attended the first meeting with Dr. James L. Tullis presiding. It was great to see so many old past-presidents again and to forget for a few hours that our backs are bent a little, our hair is sparse and white, and that a few of us need a cane to move around.

Dr. Nat Berlin stops over as our houseguest when he makes his annual trip from Miami up north, and we keep each other informed. Dr. Richard Kaplan, the current director of the Clinical Trials Cooperative Group Program at the NCI surprised me recently when he said, "You probably do not remember me, but I was one of those young clinical associates you called whippersnappers. We wore that name as a badge of honor." His 2003 budget for the Groups approaches one hundred and twenty million dollars, and for the Community Clinical Oncology Program it is forty million dollars, figures Gordon Zubrod would never have dreamed of when he initiated the program in 1956.

In a small way, I have contributed to the success of the program by chairing the myeloma and lymphoma committees in the CALGB and the breast cancer committee in SWOG. I changed the SWCCSG from a pure chemotherapy group into a multidisciplinary group and renamed the group the Southwest

Oncology Group, or SWOG as it known around the world. In addition, I stimulated the formation of the Pediatric Oncology Group (POG). The SWOG continued to thrive under the chairmanship of Dr. Charles Coltman. After Dr. Teresa Vietti stepped down as chairperson of POG, the group elected Dr. Sharon Murphy to take the reins.

After ten years in private practice, I slowed down to half days for two more years and then stopped completely in 1993. One of my last patients reminded me of the very first one I saw forty years earlier. Jean was a fifteen-year-old student when her mother brought her to the office for a consultation. She had an aggressive form of lymphoma and, because of her age, I recommended that she see Dr. Beatrice Lampkin in the highly respected Cincinnati Children's Hospital, but the mother insisted that I treat her. I gave six courses of aggressive combination chemotherapy, made her very sick, wiped out her bone marrow to the point where she needed white blood cell and platelet transfusions, made her mother miserable, and Jean responded beautifully. After she completed her treatments, I insisted that she be seen at the Children's Hospital for a second opinion about any further therapy. The doctors recommended giving four injections of methotrexate into her spinal fluid and proceeded with the first injection.

"I want you to do it," Jean cried afterwards.

"Jean, I haven't done a spinal tap in a long time."

"I don't care—you do it," she insisted.

"All right. You just do what I tell you to and it will be over in a jiffy. Sit on the edge of the table, lean on the chair. Momma, you can talk to her while I work."

Careful now, explain every little step, left index finger on the spinous process, slide the needle over the finger in the direction of the navel and feel the ever so slight give when the needle tip goes through the dura. It was just like forty years ago.

"All done."

"I told you, Mother. Didn't I tell you?" Whatever Jean said, Mother agreed. Five years later, I received an invitation to her wedding.

EPILOGUE

Oncology has come a long way since 1964, when the American Society of Clinical Oncology was founded. The driving force behind the organization was a Dutchman, Dr. Arnoldus Goudsmit, who earned his medical degree in Amsterdam in 1931. Two years later, he emigrated to the US where he studied internal medicine at the Mayo Clinic. During World War II, he was a medical officer on Iwo Jima and after the war, he practiced in Youngstown, Ohio. Goudsmit soon felt the need to exchange information and experiences with other specialists who did not turn away from treating patients with cancer. In April 1963, he and six of those physicians met to discuss "common concerns for the cancer patient." A year later, during an organizing meeting with ninety so-called chemotherapists, Goudsmit outlined the goals for a new society. That society is now known as ASCO.

Many of us did not know the word *oncology* and had to look in the dictionary to learn that *onkos* is the Greek word for mass or 'bulk.'

People used to call us cancer doctors, and now they said, "Oh, you're an 'onocologist'?"

"No, I'm an oncologist."

"That's what I said, onocologist."

With the financial support from the National Cancer Institute and the American Cancer Society, we trained thousands of young doctors to become oncologists, so many that the American Board of Internal Medicine agreed to create the new subspecialty board for Medical Oncology. Other specialties were quick to adopt the word oncology, as well. Radiotherapists became radiation oncologists and so there are surgical oncologists, GYN oncologists, and even pathology oncologists.

The mid-1950s witnessed an explosion in cancer research and cancer care, and that explosion continues today. In 1955, no physician in his right mind would have believed that acute leukemia would become a treatable disease and that today the majority of children with the disease live a normal life. The diagnosis of acute promyelocytic leukemia meant certain death in a matter of days or weeks. Now between seventy and eighty percent of patients are cured. Testicular cancer is a curable disease and so is Hodgkin's disease. However, advances in many other forms of cancer are sorely lacking. Just as the progress in surgery and radiation therapy has long slowed down to a near standstill and progress in chemotherapy has also slowed to a crawl.

How often do people not ask, "When will there be a cure for cancer?" or "Will cancer ever be cured?" I have no answer for these questions, but I do know one thing—there is no magic bullet and there will never be one. The word *cancer* is only a catch all for the numerous ways in which our bodies can go wrong somewhere. Why did one or more cells in my foot go sideways instead of going forward and not become a normal part of my body when I was a baby or a young boy? What made them do that? Why are the trillions of new cells that we make every day all perfect? Is it because our body filters out the bad ones and prevents them from multiplying? Scientists face these and many other questions every day, and the answers are exceedingly slow in coming. More funding will certainly help, but one must never forget that the puzzle is huge and that it becomes more complicated with every small step forward.

Cancer chemotherapy continues to play a major role in the treatment of cancer, as do surgery and radiation therapy, assisted by other medical specialties. The chemotherapists valued their close collaboration with pharmaceutical companies such as Eli Lilly, Lederle, Adria Laboratories in Italy, Hoffmann-La Roche in Switzerland, and Burroughs Wellcome in England. Industry leaders were genuinely interested, and both sides enjoyed our working relationship and the free exchange of information. It worked amazingly well, without the temptation of money and without oncologists being employed as the so-called advisors, consultants, or board members of today's pharmaceutical companies. Maybe *beholder* is a better word. In golf we always say, "Greed is a terrible thing," to which I would add, "I have yet to meet a good doctor who is poor."

I have few good words for those religious leaders who have moved beyond the realm of their profession and who find it necessary to extend their dictates into the spheres of politics and into our lives. If only they would convert all that energy into a softening of their hearts and devote themselves more to the ministering of the sick and dying, they and the members of their flock would once again find ways to bring understanding, acceptance and—yes—joy to our patients. Then, they may also permit stem cell research to blossom and give benefit to the patients with cancer, as well as those with an untold variety of other diseases.

Further progress in medicine can only come from basic research. A lot of work is ongoing in areas such as gene expression and the search for specific antibodies and enzymes. I read recently about an enzyme called Ras/Raf/Mek/Erk/MAP kinase and I have no idea how it works or what its importance can be. However, it does play a role somewhere in that huge cancer puzzle, and from it the next small step can be made. I am immensely grateful that in the smallest of ways I too may have helped find a tiny piece in that puzzle. It is my hope that bright young medical students and aspiring bioscientists will take our places and ensure that the fight against cancer goes on.

BIBLIOGRAPHY

Books

DeVita VT, Hellman S, Rosenberg SA, (eds): *Cancer: Principles and Practice of Oncology*, Philadelphia, JB Lippincott, 1982.

Hoogstraten B, (ed): *Cancer Research: Impact of the Cooperative Groups*, New York, Masson Publishing, 1980.

Hoogstraten B, Burn I, Bloom, HJG, (eds): *Breast Cancer*, Berlin-Heidelberg, Springer-Verlag, 1989.

Laszlo J, (ed): *The Cure of Childhood Leukemia: Into the Age of Miracles*, New Brunswick, Rutgers University Press, 1996.

Snapper I, Turner LB, Moscovitz HL: *Multiple Myeloma*, New York, Grune, 1953.

Tuchman BW: *A Distant Mirror: The Calamitous 14th Century*, New York, Knopf, 1978.

Zubrod CG: *Stairway of Surprise*, Baltimore, Gateway Press, 1997.

Articles and Chapters

Broughan TA, Esselstyn CB, Jr.: Indications for and techniques of limited breast surgery. In Hoogstraten B, Burn I, Bloom HJG, (eds): Breast Cancer, pp 161–167, Berlin-Heidelberg, Springer-Verlag, 1989.

Crewdson J: "Fraud in breast cancer study: Doctor gave phony data over twelve years," *Chicago Tribune*, March 13, 1994.

Crile GW: An analysis of 1,347 cases of malignant tumors of the breast with special reference to management and end-result, Lancet 1:1–12, 1931.

DeVita VT: The relationship between tumor mass and resistance to chemotherapy, *Cancer* 51: 1209–1220, 1983.

Duckett JW: The Halsted heritage, *Surgery* 55: 859–869, 1964.

Farber S: Toward the control of cancer, Second Annual David A. Karnofsky Memorial Lecture, *Cancer* 28: 856–861, 1971.

Gelhorn A: Invited remarks on the current status of research in clinical cancer chemotherapy, *Cancer Chemotherapy Reports* 5: 1–12, 1959.

Gilman A, Philips FS: The biological actions and therapeutic applications of the B-chloroethyl amines and sulfides, *Science* 103:409–415, 1946.

Gilman A: The initial clinical trial of nitrogen mustard, *Am J Surgery* 105: 574–578, 1963.

Haagensen CD, Stout AP: Disorders of the Breast. In Christopher F, (ed): *A Textbook of Surgery*, pp 808–837, Philadelphia, WB Saunders, 1952.

Haddow A: Thoughts on chemical therapy, David A. Karnofsky Memorial Lecture, *Cancer* 26: 737–754, 1970.

Holland JF: Who should treat acute leukemia? *JAMA* 209:1511–1513, 1969.

Holland JF: *E Pluribus Unum*, Presidential Address, *Cancer Research* 31: 1319–1329, 1971.

Holland JF: Breaking the cure barrier, Karnofsky Memorial Lecture, *J Clinical Oncology* 1: 71–90, 1983.

Jacobson LO et al: Nitrogen mustard therapy, *JAMA* 132: 263–271, 1946.

Knox R: The Harvard fraud case: Where does the problem lie? Medical News, *JAMA* 249: 1797–1807, 1983.

McBride G: The Sloan-Kettering affair: Could it have happened anywhere? Medical News, *JAMA* 229: 1398–1410, 1974.

Soignet SL et al: Complete remission after treatment of acute promyelocytic leukemia with arsenic trioxide, *New Engl J Med* 339: 1341–1348, 1998.

Sun HD, Ma L, Hu X-C, Zhang P, Chin J: Arsenic trioxide in the treatment of acute promyelocytic leukemia, *Integrat Chin West Med* 12: 170–172, 1992.

Wooldridge Committee Report to the President. Biochemical Science and its Administration. A study of the National Institutes of Health, Washington, US Government Print Office, 1965

Zhang P, Wang SY, Hu, YH: Arsenic trioxide treated 72 cases of acute promyelocytic leukemia, *Chin J Hem* 17: 58–62, 1996.

Zubrod CG et al: The chemotherapy program of the National Cancer Institute: History, analysis, and plans, *Cancer Chemotherapy Reports* 50: 349–380, 1966.

Zubrod CG: The basis for progress in chemotherapy, *Cancer* 30: 1474–1479, 1972.

ABOUT THE AUTHOR

Born in Holland, Barth Hoogstraten emigrated to the United States in 1956. He was a professor of medicine at the Mount Sinai School of Medicine in New York City and in 1970 became the first American Cancer Society Professor of Clinical Oncology at the University of Kansas. He chaired the Committee on Combination Chemotherapy of the National Breast Cancer Task Force, represented the United States as a member of the Committee on the Current Treatment of Cancer of the International Union against Cancer (1982–1993), and he was chairman of the Southwest Oncology Group (1972–1981). Hoogstraten was the recipient of an international fellowship from the Fogarty International Center. He was also elected a Fellow of The Royal Society of Medicine.

978-0-595-36010-9
0-595-36010-6

www.ingramcontent.com/pod-product-compliance
Lightning Source LLC
Chambersburg PA
CBHW020744180526
45163CB00001B/339